P9-BYK-380

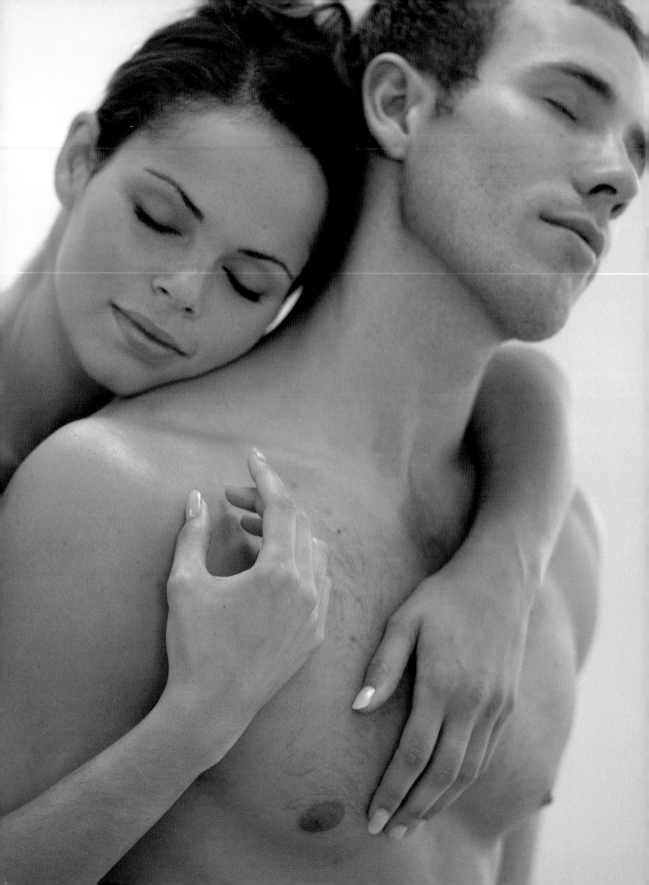

ANNE HOOPER

Erotic Massage

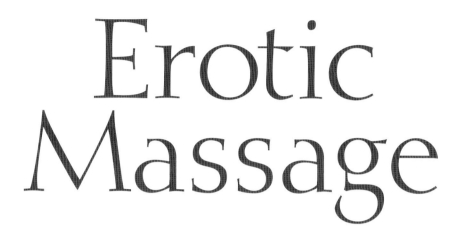

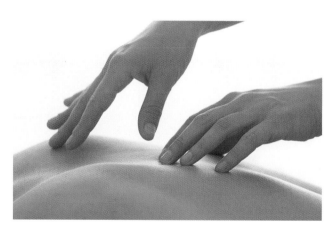

enrich your lovemaking
through the power of touch

LONDON, NEW YORK, MUNICH, MELBOURNE, DELHI

TO KENNETH RAY STUBBS, AN INSPIRED TEACHER

Brand Manager for Anne Hooper Lynne Brown
Senior Art Editor Helen Spencer
Designer Philip Lord
Book Editor Phil Hunt
Senior Editor Peter Jones
US Editor Margaret Parrish
DTP Designers Karen Constanti, Jackie Plant, Traci Salter
Production Sarah Sherlock

Art Director Carole Ash
Publishing Director Corinne Roberts

First published in the United States in 2005 by DK Publishing, Inc.
375 Hudson Street, New York, New York 10014

00 01 02 03 04 05 06 07 08 09 10 9 8 7 6 5 4 3 2 1

Copyright © 2005 Dorling Kindersley Limited
Text copyright © 2005 Anne Hooper

All rights reserved under International and Pan-American Copyright Conventions.
No part of this publication may be reproduced, stored in a retrieval system, or
transmitted in any form or by any means, electronic, mechanical, photocopying, recording,
or otherwise, without the prior written permission of the copyright owner.

A catalog record for this book is available from the Library of Congress.
ISBN 0-7566-0526-1

Color Reproduction by GRB Editrice
Printed and bound in Singapore by Tien Wah Press

See our complete product line at
www.dk.com

Contents

Introduction 6

Making contact 8

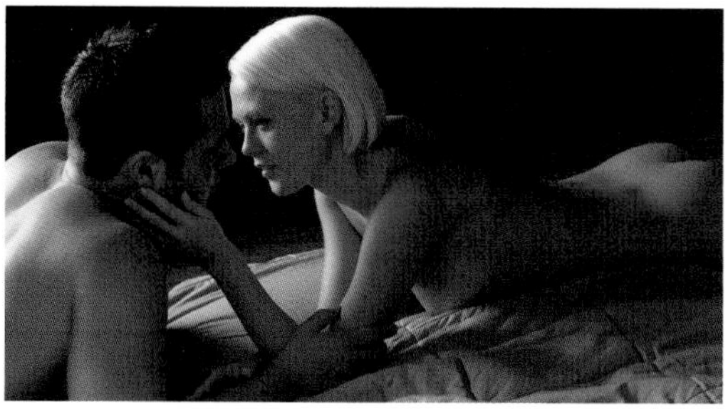

In the bedroom 42

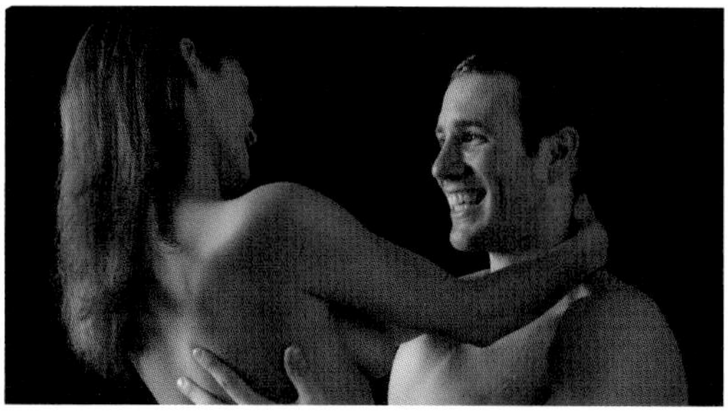

Sensual massage 70

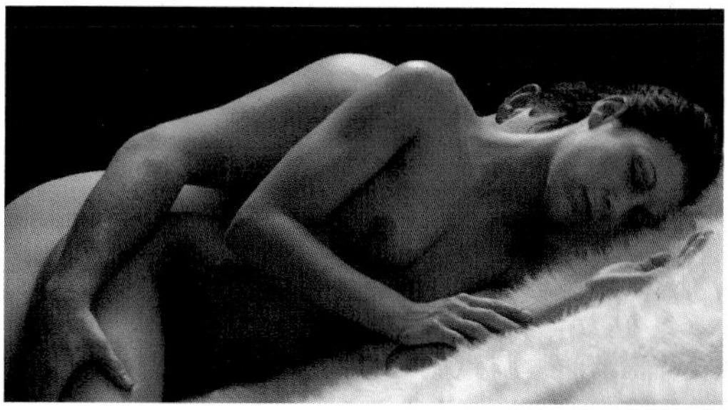

Intimate massage 106

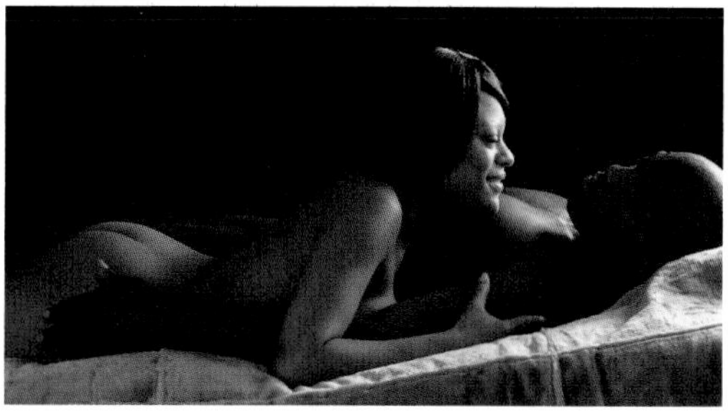

Self-touch techniques 122

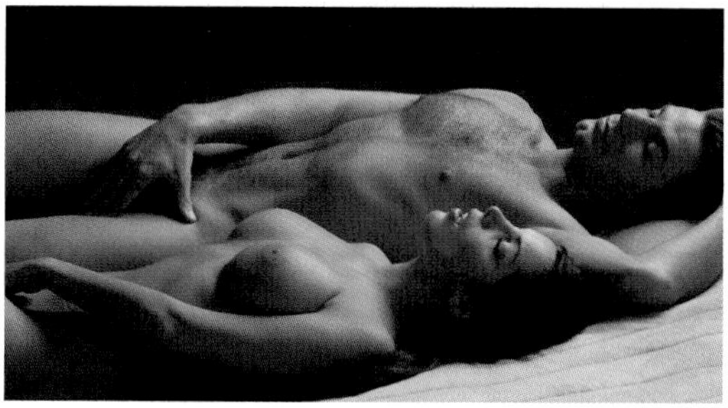

Touch for life changes 136

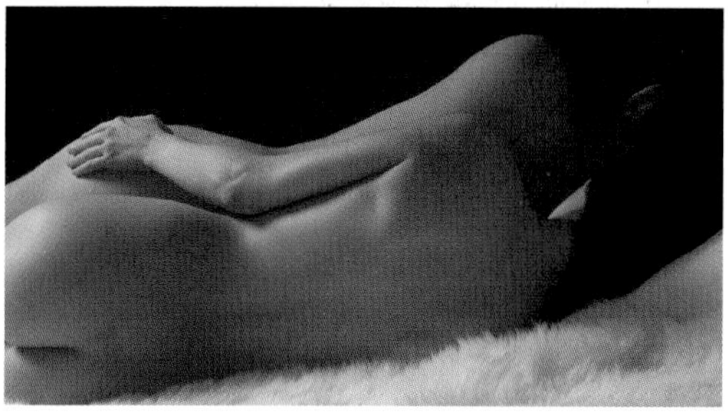

Index 158

Acknowledgments 160

Introduction

Sensual touch is one of the greatest gifts in the world. What's more, it's not difficult to learn. A sexy massage done by a wonderful, tactile partner has the ability to light up the entire body. Your body takes on a rosy hue and so does your mood!

My first serious exposure to sensual massage was at the hands of a massage trainer teaching students at the then newly formed Institute for the Advanced Study of Human Sexuality in San Francisco. This was the first American organization licensed to award a degree in sexology. And Kenneth Ray Stubbs, the teacher, was the closest you can get to being a trainer of genius. For years afterward I went to his sensual massage training courses whenever the opportunity arose.

"One of the first things I learned was to feel completely comfortable with nudity. It's a prerequisite for good massage."

I have referred to his methods, techniques, fantasy approach, and sensational touch constantly in my books. I learned so much from him. Thank you Ray.

The Institute, while encouraging important research work and serious theses from its students, also included a great deal of "bodywork" among students. One of the first things I learned was to feel completely comfortable with nudity. It's a prerequisite for good massage. If you, the masseur/se can't feel comfortable, just how would you expect the person you are massaging to do so?

In fact, my first meeting with Ray Stubbs went as follows: I was being ushered across the foyer of the Institute by the founder, the Rev. Ted McIlvenna, when a door burst open on the left and out flocked a troupe of glowing, laughing people, all completely nude. At their head, carrying a bowl of soapy water, was a tall, thin young man with a generous moustache. "Anne. Meet Ray," Ted said. Ray shifted the bowl to one hand and without any self-consciousness of any kind, solemnly shook hands with the other.

It was my first lesson in how lack of inhibition fosters feelings of comfort. As I greeted him I thought the situation wonderful. It never occurred to me that this might be in any way uncongenial. It was the complete opposite. Ray and his students had just ended a terrific massage training session and the waves of well-being emanating from their rosy bodies, made me long to join in the studies.

It's thanks to Ray's brilliant teaching that I want to pass on the fabulous present of sensual massage. It's one of the best things in the world. So please—give it a try.

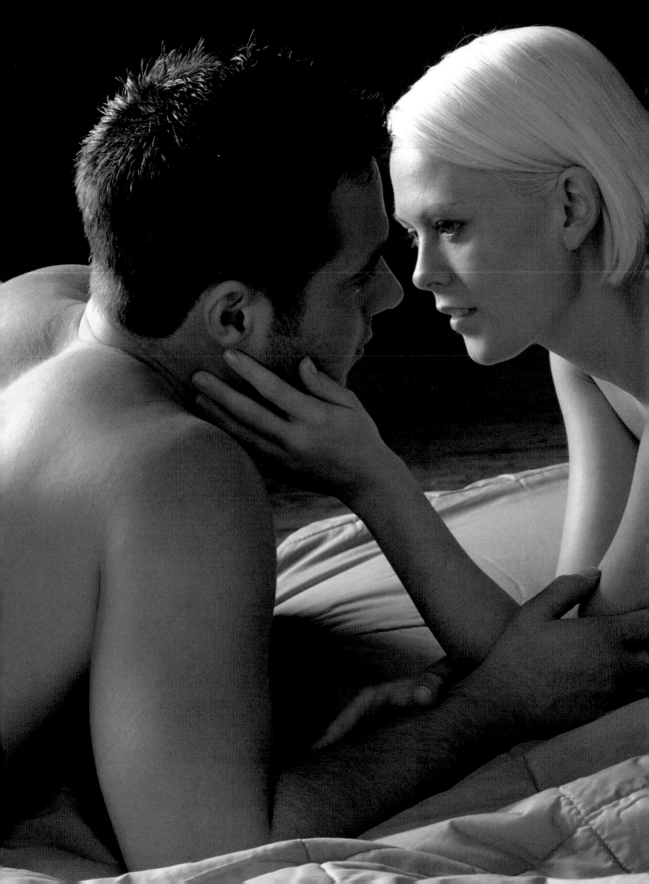

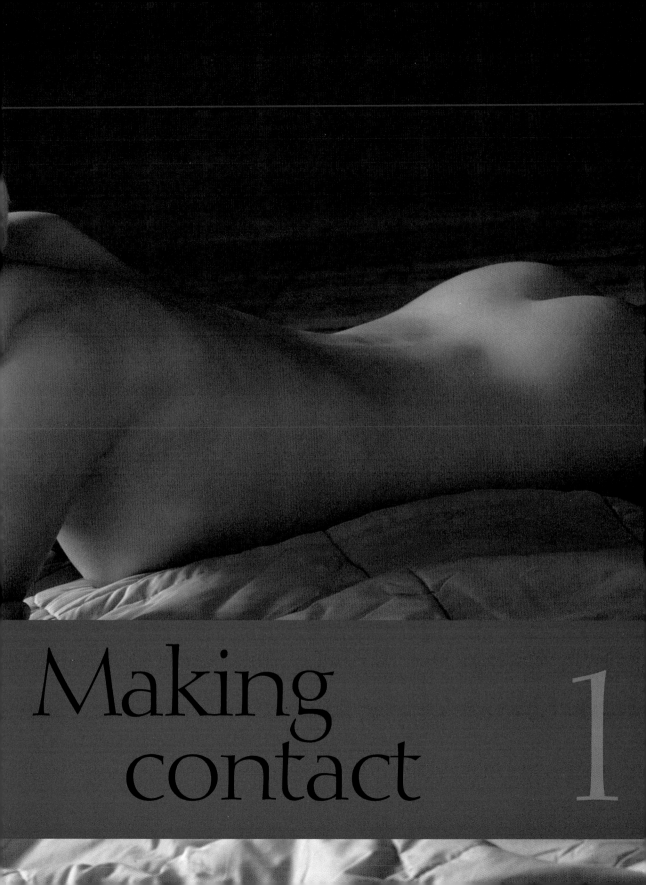

Making contact

1

Each other's skin

Most of us fail to give our skin a second thought. It's just there—the covering that protects the inner flesh from the outside air. Yet the skin is a human being's biggest sex organ, and it also provides us with a direct route to each other's emotions.

If we are excited or sad, angry or hopeful, the emotions will surface when our lovers lay hands on us. This is because a basic type of sensuality is planted within us when we are babies. What that sensuality consists of depends on the quality of touch we received when we were tiny. If that touch was good, our maturing feelings will grow into a happy enjoyment of sensuality, but if it was bad, our adult response to touch will probably become aggressive rejection.

Relationship problems

A more complicated problem emerges when you have been in a sexual relationship for some time—perhaps it has been successful in terms of orgasms but the lack of passion leaves you disappointed. Neither you nor your partner has yet worked out that passion has everything to do with how we give and receive touch. Touch isn't just a matter of hands on bodies; it's also a state of mind. By awakening our early memories, we may be able to expand the spiritual side of touch.

The "up" side of connecting through touch is that it acts as a shortcut to a person's innermost sensual character. Anna said of her new lover: "I'd known David for years, as a friend—a nice, trustworthy, dull friend. Shortly after my marriage broke up he took me out to dinner so I could cry on his shoulder—which I did. But after the meal, he held my hand when we walked to the car and I felt as though an electric current were surging through me. I could suddenly feel things about his sensuality, and therefore about him, that I'd had no idea existed."

"Four years later, he still needs only to touch me and I'm instantly connected to this marvelous inner man. It's truly exciting, knowing that such an intensely sensual human being is wrapped up in this seemingly ordinary exterior."

SKIN SENSITIVITY

Some areas are more sensitive than others because they contain more nerve endings, very closely packed together. For instance, the fingertips, where the nerves are densely packed, are much more sensitive to touch than the skin of the back.

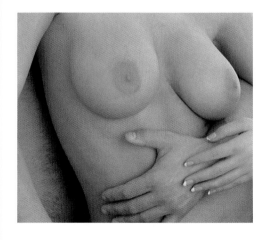

Loving touch

The feelings of warmth and intimacy engendered by tender, loving touch will help your relationship to grow deeper and stronger.

Cultural differences

European men and women touch each other conspicuously more than their North American counterparts. A touch survey showed that American friends touched two to three times an hour while Europeans touched on average 100 times an hour. Our culture, therefore, and even literally the land we are born into, will affect our attitudes to touch and our experiences of it. Where touch may offer Europeans feelings of security, Americans could feel threatened by it. Establishing your good intentions at the start of a relationship may turn out to be far more important in the US than in, for example, France. Which isn't to say that good intentions aren't always important—they are. Getting these across before laying a loving finger on a potential partner is a practical rule of thumb!

I hope I've made the case for finding out about your partner's first experiences of touch and the role of touch in his or her early family life. This is the sort of information that will allow your relationship to expand mentally and emotionally while your skin—and that of your partner—becomes increasingly responsive to wonderful touch sensation.

"Touch brings with it memories. In order to enjoy wonderful touch with a partner now, it helps to know what touch meant to that partner when he or she was a baby. Gaining an understanding of our own touch histories is also a good idea."

Exploration

When exploring each other's bodies, you are helping to build mutual trust while giving and receiving sensual pleasure.

THE TOUCH QUESTIONNAIRE

You and your partner can find out about each other's experience of touch in infancy and childhood by working through the Touch Questionnaire below. The questions are aimed at stirring the memory and providing you with hitherto stored information. Remember that there are no right or wrong answers.

Infancy

- What are your earliest recollections of being lovingly touched?
- What are your earliest recollections of being punishingly touched?
- What are your earliest recollections of touching someone?
- What are your first memories of sensual feeling?
- Which member or members of your family hugged you regularly?
- Did you have a security blanket or other comfort object as a baby?

- What are your earliest recollections of the textures you slept in?
- What are your earliest recollections of the textures you were clothed in?

Childhood

- Did you sleep alone or with someone?
- If you slept with someone, what do you remember of physical contact?
- Did you play touch games as a child?
- If you did, what was your parents' attitude toward this?
- Did you caress yourself as a child?
- If you did, what was your parents' attitude toward this?
- Were you physically close to your best friends?
- If you were, what attitude did others take to this?
- As a child, did you hug your parents?
- Did they hug you?
- How old were you when this stopped?

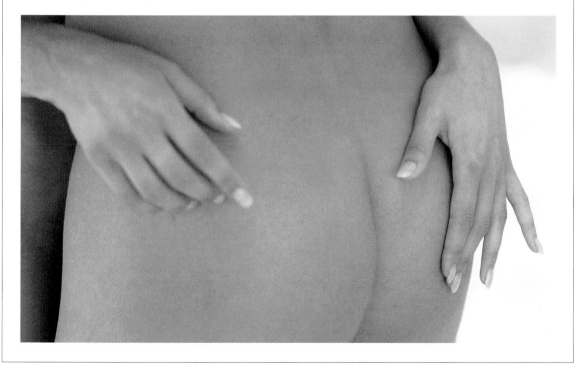

The early stages

Part of the natural life "task" of adolescents is to separate from their parents in order to become independent beings. They need to accomplish this both for their own sakes and for those of their parents. As part of this separation, the hugs and caresses between parents and child usually stop. This then means that the young person craves sensual input.

The reason children withdraw physically from their parents is the burgeoning of sexual feeling. Their biological clocks send a flood of sex hormones into the bloodstream, and touch that was previously sensual now begins to have a sexual element in it. Loving touch suddenly needs to be directed toward a lover, or at least someone who has the potential to be a lover.

For example, your partner may be afraid to reveal crucial details of his or her early life because they include an episode of abuse or even incest. To help offload these distressing recollections, your partner may need to hear you say you will not be disgusted or repelled by

Listen and respond

When you are learning about a new partner's sensual history, listen to what he or she has to say and respond to it.

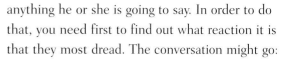

anything he or she is going to say. In order to do that, you need first to find out what reaction it is that they most dread. The conversation might go:

You: "What is it that scares you most?"

Partner: "I'm afraid you'll think I'm awful, that you won't like me anymore."

You: "I promise you that you won't shock me, that nothing you can say will make me dislike you, and that if you're going to feel bad I'll do everything I can to make you feel better."

A word of warning: You need to examine your intentions before making these promises, because having made them, you've got to stick to them. If you think that you can't follow through, you should refrain from promising. Indeed, this would be the time to call a halt to the proceedings because your partner could be deeply upset were you to let him or her down.

A partner's distress

Your permission to disclose might unleash a storm. For example, it can be very moving to talk about an episode of abuse, which perhaps has never been brought out before. Be prepared to do a great deal of sympathizing, comforting, and just listening. It might be necessary to delay the rest of the exercise until another occasion.

If your partner, having revealed a deep secret, is distressed and cannot recover, and you feel that you are out of your depth, continue to be warm and supportive but help him or her find a professional counselor to consult as soon as possible. Encourage your partner to go for this assistance, offer to go along with him or her as well if that seems like a good idea, and offer support while he or she tries to come to terms with this negative experience.

Touch play

One of the joyous aspects of falling in love
is the rediscovery of the child within us.
Suddenly it feels right to laugh, play,
flirt, and provoke. It's a wonderful way
to discover what spontaneity and life
our lover draws from within us.

As real children, of course, we play too, for the same reasons and with the same results. We learn about the world and the people around us, and touch plays a huge part in this education.

Even if we weren't deliberately massaged as babies, most of us learned to enjoy touch while we were being handled, bounced, petted, cuddled, and caressed—but not all. Some of us, with cold, undemonstrative parents, were deprived of this vital start.

Learning positive responses

Knowledge of touch, which seems obvious to those of us who were fortunate enough to have had sensual parents, won't exist in the minds of those who were play- and skin-starved.

The good news is that even if we haven't had too much good touching as infants, we can still take in good touch at a later age. Indeed, this can go further. By learning positive responses to being touched, we can actually develop new neural pathways in the brain and catch up on experiencing good sensuality. So embarking on a series of touch games is a way of feeding information into our brains

that we can use when appropriate. We can expand our knowledge and our range of sensual experience in this way.

Tuning in to moods

Different kinds of touch suit different kinds of occasions. If a friend's parent has just died, it is fine to hold him or her and offer comfort with your physical presence, but it would not be appropriate to suggest stripping off for a sensual massage. And someone who is very angry will be irritated if you suggest playing touch games. So always take the time to find out how your friend is feeling. But note that massage can be highly beneficial, emotionally as well as physically.

SOCIALIZING EFFECTS

We now know, through work with autistic children, that it is possible to introduce a human being to touch experience in order to change his or her perception of the world. The logical conclusion is that we may still be able to socialize unruly adults with some intense touch experience. So being kissed, hugged, and stroked as babies is vital to how responsive as partners we are in later life.

Love and play

It is no accident that partners play together at the beginning of a new love affair—it is through play that we learn. Play teaches us about ourselves, our emotions and those of our partner, and how relationships function through interactions. In other words, we get to know each other.

Benefits of touch

Many people have benefited greatly from being introduced (or reintroduced) to the experience of touch, particularly in the form of massage. I remember one young woman in a women's group who was severely depressed. Letting herself be touched in the group massage, and discovering how comforting this felt, was her starting point for recovery. The warm, nonthreatening physical contact helped her to feel valued and less isolated. This then increased her self-esteem and self-confidence, which gave her new hope for the future.

Even those of us who did get a lot of play and tumble as babies can still forget the value of touch. But it can be fun to be reminded of it, and for those of us who were starved of touch, massage is a terrific way of catching up on the good sensations we have missed.

Getting close

Touch conveys love, reassurance, comfort, and, above all, appreciation.

Loving expression

Eye contact, smiles, and gentle, loving touch help you express your feelings for each other.

STRESS RELIEF

The symptoms of stress often include muscular tension. By relaxing the muscles, massage helps the mind to relax and so helps to create a feeling of contentment.

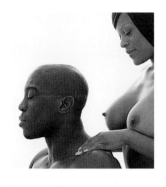

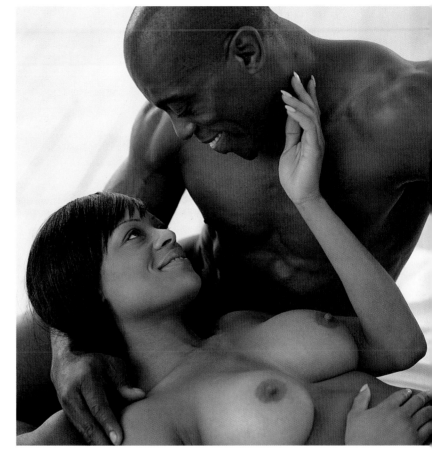

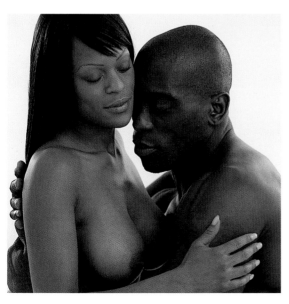

"It's always worth remembering that a massage is a sensuous experience for the person giving it as well as for the recipient."

Value of touch

It's wise to appreciate the sensuality of touch for its own sake and not to view it merely as a preliminary to the physical act of sex.

Agreeing on the rules

Many readers of this book will be in established relationships that they want to extend. They will already have grown comfortable with nudity and will also have made the leap from sensual touch to sexual intercourse. In theory, then, they will possess a wealth of sensual information about each other.

Not all students of sensual touch, however, are yet living together or married, and there will be some who are just beginning a relationship. These are men and women who are hoping to set that new friendship off on a sensual footing, and who will be gathering sensual facts about each other along the way.

Establishing ground rules

At the beginning of the first massage session, discuss the boundaries of the massage. You might tell your partner that sexual intercourse is not part of the proceedings, that verbal feedback between the two of you is expected, and that if at any time the massagee dislikes something, he or she has only to say so for it to stop. The person who is giving the massage also has the option of withdrawing from the session.

The versatile massage

One of the delights of massage is that it can be used in a variety of ways and at different levels of intimacy, combining physical and emotional pleasure.

BASIC MASSAGE GUIDELINES

- Perform the massage on a firm bed or on the floor, and cover it with soft towels for your comfort and to protect it from the massage oil
- If you are wearing clothes when giving a massage, they should be comfortable and should not impede your movements
- Make sure your hands are clean and your nails are short with no jagged edges
- Ask your partner to tell you whether or not the strokes you are using are enjoyable
- Despite the pleasure it gives, there are times when massage is inadvisable. Do not massage over varicose veins or recent scar tissue
- Do not massage if you or your partner has a skin infection, a fever, a contagious illness, thrombosis, phlebitis, or heart problems
- Do not massage if you or your partner has recently undergone surgery, has suffered serious injury, or has acute pain
- Do not massage if you or your partner has any severe swelling or bruising, or acute inflammation

If in doubt, always seek medical advice.

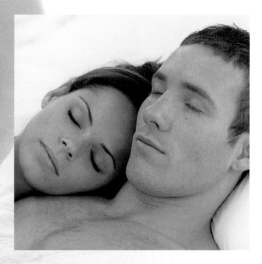

Beginning the massage

Massage is a more structured activity than getting to know a friend. Making the introductory moves into a deliberate ritual allows them to become more acceptable and gives each of you the opportunity to feel comfortable about touching. When you are going to give a massage, always lay out in advance any equipment you need and keep the lights dim.

Preparation

Start by carrying out a simple ceremony. Sit cross-legged in front of each other, without touching, and practice deep breathing in unison. Breathe in through the nose for a count of four, and then out through the mouth for a count of four. Do this for five minutes. Then, each of you perform the exercises on pages 24–25.

SENSUAL SURROUNDINGS

A massage is a sensual experience, so the surroundings should emphasize sensuality. The skin tenses when it is cold and is likely to experience touch as painful. When the skin is warm, the whole body relaxes and touch is experienced as pleasure. You must therefore ensure that the room is very warm and that your massaging hands are, too.

Clothing

For the person giving the massage, loose, light clothing, affording maximum movement and a sense of freedom, is ideal. Take off any rings and other jewelry you might be wearing, because these can catch on your partner's skin or hair.

Cleanliness

Scrupulous cleanliness is important, and clean hands are essential because even a tiny grain of dirt on the hand can be experienced as a piece of sharp grit when it is rubbed over the skin during massage. If you are the one giving the massage, wash your hands in hot water before you begin. Then rub warm massage oil into your hands. Apply a liberal coating to the area of your partner's skin you are going to massage.

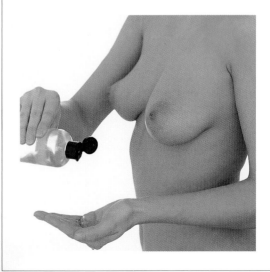

EXERCISE ROUTINE

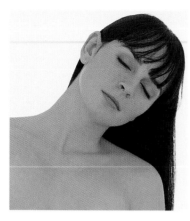

1 Rotate head

For a count of three, rotate your head slowly from side to side, extending it forward then backward so that the bones in your neck are loosened.

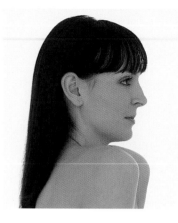

2 Rotate shoulders

Then, for a count of four, rotate both shoulders at the same time, first forward and then backward, stretching them as far as they will go in each direction so that they loosen up and the arm sockets feel exercised.

3 Stretch arms

Next, stretch your arms out in front of you as far as they will go, with the backs of the hands facing each other.

4 Circle arms

Windmill your arms slowly in circles, stretching as far back as you can reach while turning them so that the palms of the hands are now facing completely outward.

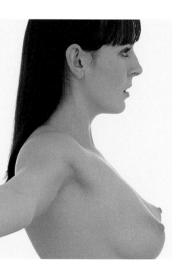

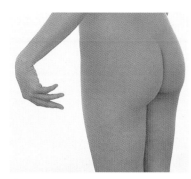

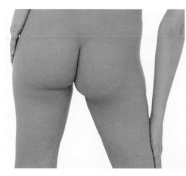

5 Rotate hands

Now rotate your hands so that the wrist bones are exercised, wriggling your fingers to loosen them at the same time. Do this quickly, for a count of 10.

6 Stretch

Then stretch down from the waist to the floor, first to the left, then to the right, as if you were trying to touch the floor. This exercises the muscles at the side of the waist and stretches the spine in the pelvic girdle.

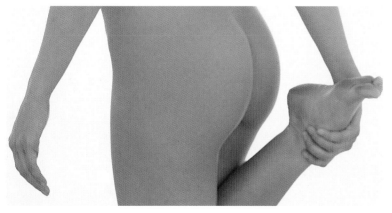

7 Leg stretch

Standing on one leg and holding on to something for support, take hold of the ankle and draw the heel up toward the buttock; then stretch it out in front of you several times. Exercise first one leg, then the other, to tone up the muscles and exercise the knee joints. To exercise your ankle joints, stand on one leg, point the other in front of you, and rotate the

foot first clockwise and then counter-clockwise. Repeat the exercise on the other foot, each time for a count of 10.

8 Face muscles

Finally, exercise the muscles of your face. Screw it up as hard as possible, grimacing to stretch your mouth. Hold for a count of five, and then let go and relax.

RELAXING TOGETHER

Lie side by side, flat on your backs, and make a conscious effort to relax. This may be difficult if either of you is not used to it, or is feeling self-conscious. To help you relax, try to empty your minds of any intrusive thoughts, and breathe slowly and deeply.

Then, using the tense/relax exercise, work your way through your limbs once more, this time focusing on muscle tension. To do this simple exercise, exaggerate the tension in each limb in turn by clenching the muscles for a count of three. Let go and relax for a further count of three. When you feel your body is fully relaxed, lie still and rest for about five minutes.

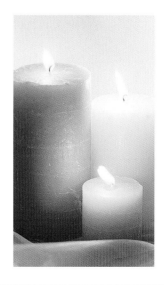

Massage games

In California, where I did some of my sex therapy training, most therapists use simple touch games to help their clients relax and become more intimate. Here is a series of massage games that are nonsexual, nonthreatening, and fun.

The famous Indian sex manual, the *Kama Sutra*, makes frequent reference to shampooing. This was a type of massage service provided to wealthy Indian men by eunuchs, and by women of low caste who were also valued for their sexual services. In Ancient India, shampooing was a skilled craft, and it is on this sensuous art that the pleasurable touch game shown on pages 28–29 is based.

CLOSING THE THIRD EYE

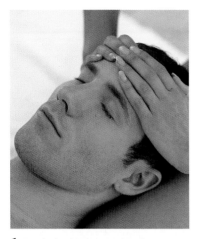

1 Begin by resting your palms on either side of your partner's head, with your fingertips meeting at the "third eye." Hold your hands there for a minute or two of light yet enclosing touch.

2 Then place your right palm on your partner's forehead, put your left palm on top of it, and press down firmly but gently, with gradually increasing pressure, for about 10 seconds. Release slowly, eventually lifting your palms from the forehead. Repeat the stroke several times.

Preparation

The "third eye" exercise is a wonderful starter to any session of massage games, and it consists of gentle strokes that concentrate on the "third eye," the energy center on the forehead above the nose and the gap between the eyebrows. Your partner lies face up, and you kneel at his or her head.

The sensual shampoo

This is ideally performed with your friend or partner sitting up, and leaning back with head tilted back over the end of a chair or of a bathtub, preferably with adequate padding between the chair (or bathtub) and the neck. The ground below should be covered with towels and a bowl in which to catch the overflow.

Stand at the side of your friend and, after dampening (not soaking) the hair, apply enough of a mild shampoo to produce lather that will slide through the hair comfortably but not run off in rivulets. The secret to achieving this is to use water sparingly, adding to it only if necessary. Then give your partner a sensuous, massaging shampoo.

Some people won't want to bother with drying their hair after the massage and may prefer the almost identical dry version, as shown on the right.

DRY SHAMPOOING

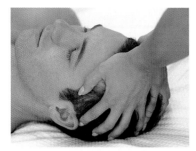

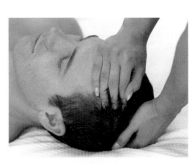

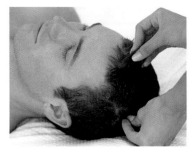

1 Using both hands, massage your partner's scalp lightly with your fingertips for several minutes, moving your fingertips over the scalp in small circles.

2 Support your partner's head with one hand or, if you prefer, lean it against your body. Then cup your other hand on top of the head and gently rotate the scalp.

3 Take small locks of your partner's hair between the thumb and forefinger of each hand. Pull each lock gently to create pricklings of sensation in your partner's scalp.

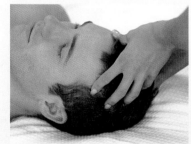

4 Now massage the scalp again, this time using your fingertips, instead of a cupped hand, to move it around in small circles. Be careful not to snag the hair.

The dress-maker's dummy

In this, our first whole-body exercise, one partner lends his or her body as a completely passive object for the other to manipulate. This means, of course, that the lender must be assured that nothing will be done that could hurt or injure.

Head tilting

Begin by standing behind him. Take his head in both hands. Gently tilt it from side to side, then backward and forward. Don't force any movement—stop when the body resists your touch.

As the name suggests, in this touch game the partner who is taking the passive role is treated as if he or she were an inanimate object. When playing the part of the dummy, each of you will find that there can be great pleasure in feeling helpless. The game takes place in two parts: in the first, the man is the dummy, and in the second, the woman takes that role.

Standing up

For the first stage of his turn as the dummy, the man should stand up straight and make no movements. The woman's job is to experiment with her partner's versatility of movement, tilting and rotating his head and arms into a variety of positions. He may keep his clothes on, as long as they are not constricting, but he should take his shoes off. To get started, try the following moves.

The woman stands behind her partner and begins by gently rotating his head and tilting it from side to side and backward and forward (*see left*). She then slips both hands under her partner's armpits and pulls up briefly to take some of the weight off his feet.

Now, the woman focuses on her partner's arms. First, she should take his right hand in her right hand and shake it up and down, gently at first and then more vigorously; after this, shake it from side to side, again increasing in vigor.

Next, one arm at a time, the woman should hold his hand in her right hand, then put her left hand on the lower part of his arm and use it to turn the arm as far to the left, then right, as possible. Finally, she should bend and pull her partner's arms, and rotate his lower arms in large circles, first clockwise, then counterclockwise.

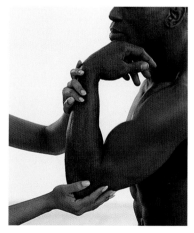

Bending the arm
Hold his right elbow with your right hand. With your left hand, bend his lower arm up against his upper arm so it is doubled up. Then exert a firm pressure with both hands. Hold for a count of three, let go, and repeat.

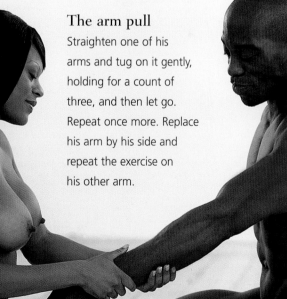

The arm pull
Straighten one of his arms and tug on it gently, holding for a count of three, and then let go. Repeat once more. Replace his arm by his side and repeat the exercise on his other arm.

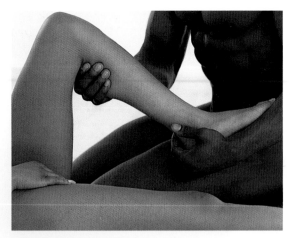

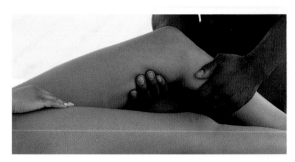

The legs

Repeat all the arm movements, this time on each leg in turn. Remember to use firm but gentle pressure when you are manipulating the limbs.

Leg care

Don't be afraid of lifting your partner's limbs, but make sure that you do not twist them into uncomfortable positions or jerk too hard on them.

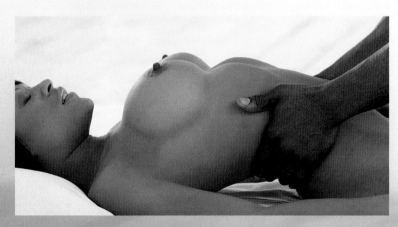

The waist lift

Kneel over your "dummy," lean down, put your arms around her waist, then pull her up toward you to arch her back. Hold for a count of three before lowering her back to the ground. Do not attempt this movement if your partner is heavy.

"When you are the dummy, stay passive and make no attempt to 'help' by moving an arm or leg."

Lying down

The second stage of the game takes place with the dummy lying down. The man's job is still the same: that of playing with his partner's limbs to see what shapes he can make with her. If the woman is particularly tiny and light, the man may like to lower her gently to the ground by standing behind her and supporting her weight with his arms under her armpits.

The sensuous foot

Feet are notoriously ticklish extremities. Many people can't bear for them to be touched at all or are insistent that a foot massage will do nothing for them. But it's worth stopping to think why the foot should be so ticklish.

According to reflexology theory, the foot plays a major role within the body's nervous system: every nerve in the foot (and there are many thousands) is connected up with a corresponding nerve somewhere else in the body. If you visualize every nerve in the body packed into your foot, you will get an insight into why the foot is so sensitive.

Foot massage

Equip yourself with a couple of warm, fluffy towels, some warmed massage oil, and a box of tissues in case of spills. Before beginning the massage, wash your partner's feet thoroughly in warm water and dry them. Then firmly—not lightly in case of ticklishness—coat the foot with oil.

Use the strokes shown on pages 36–37. When you have finished massaging one foot, gently lower it to the ground, wrap it in a towel, and perform the same procedure on the other foot.

Reflexology

Reflexologists believe that when you massage the foot, you are also, in effect, massaging the rest of the body, sending bolts of sensation and therefore energy throughout the nervous system.

"My partner likes to begin by gently caressing my lower shin down to my toes; it feels exquisite."

Knuckling

Hold the foot with your left hand and press your right knuckles hard into the sole. Cover the entire sole with small circling movements.

Thumbing

Work over the whole area of the sole with both thumbs simultaneously. Circle them slowly with as deep a pressure as possible.

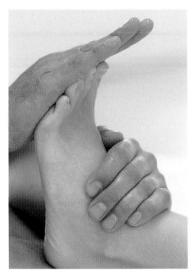

Bending the toes

Press the toes forward, for a count of 10, as if you were trying to bend them in the wrong direction. Repeat this three times.

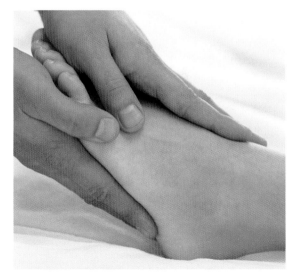

Circling

Massage the top of the foot with your thumbs, applying moderate pressure. When you near the ankle, circle with your fingertips and avoid the ankle bone itself—always avoid massaging directly on a bone.

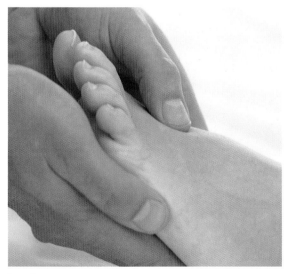

In the grooves

The top of the foot is divided by raised tendons with grooves between them. Support the foot with one hand and, pressing firmly, run the tip of your thumb down these grooves from ankle to toe.

Finishing off

Hold the foot between your hands and imagine that they are beaming energy into it. Then, very slowly, slide your hands away from the foot, pausing for a very long time before finally letting go.

Playful moves

When I was taught sensual massage, I was amazed to find that we started it with a bath. It was from this and other relaxation rituals I learned that I gathered a variety of ideas which I've adapted to be enjoyed specifically by lovers.

The starting point to a massage session (and to some lovemaking sessions, of course) can be a warm dip. Floating in the bathtub may bring back subconscious memories of floating deep inside our mothers' wombs—the most complete sensual experience we will ever know—where we are enclosed by sensation. After bathing, dry each other with warm, fluffy towels. You can

The hair sweep

Let your hair hang down loosely onto his naked skin and sweep and flick it erotically over his body and limbs.

then begin a massage, make love, or simply indulge in affectionate touching such as playing with each other's hair, hugging, cuddling, kissing, and stroking each other.

Playing with hair

If one or both of you has long hair, playing with it can be a subtly erotic experience. Long-haired individuals can try the curiously tantalizing hair sweep. One partner (usually the man) lies flat and the long-haired one (usually the woman) covers his naked body with her hair, dragging it across the skin, sweeping it, and flicking it backward and forward. For those of you with short locks, simply taking time to wash and brush each other's hair can also be delightful, and is a subtle method of getting close.

The magic mirror

This self-help exercise can help you overcome inhibitions and involves simply looking at yourself naked in a mirror and talking about which parts of your body you like and which you dislike. You could look in the mirror while brushing your partner's hair, and then reveal some of your feelings about your appearance.

WARMING OIL

To warm up your massage oil before you begin, stand or lean the bottle in a bowl of hot water for a few minutes.

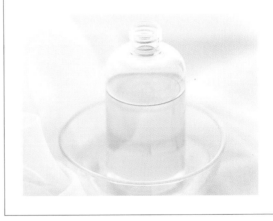

Hugging and cuddling

Don't be afraid of hugging
and cuddling. Spend hours,
days, even weeks on these
pleasing activities, if
that feels right.

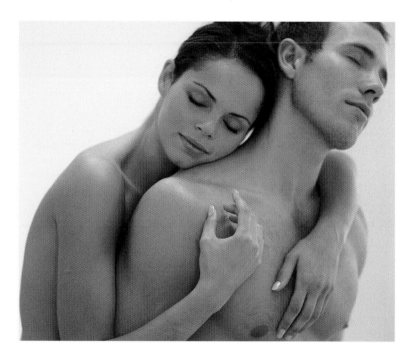

Body strokes

Take the initiative in running your hands lightly all over your partner's body, stroking it with the backs and tips of your fingers.

Touching hands

Touch and caress each other's hands, stroking them, fitting them into shapes together, massaging them, and lifting and kissing them.

"After bathing, you can begin a massage, make love, or simply indulge in affectionate touching such as playing with each other's hair, hugging, cuddling, kissing, and stroking each other."

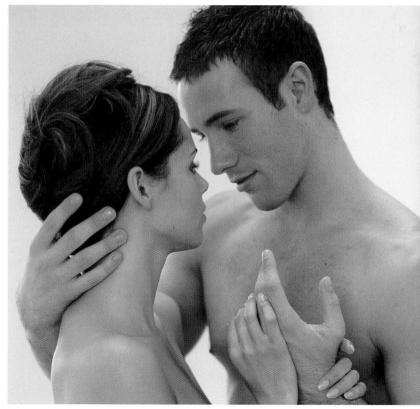

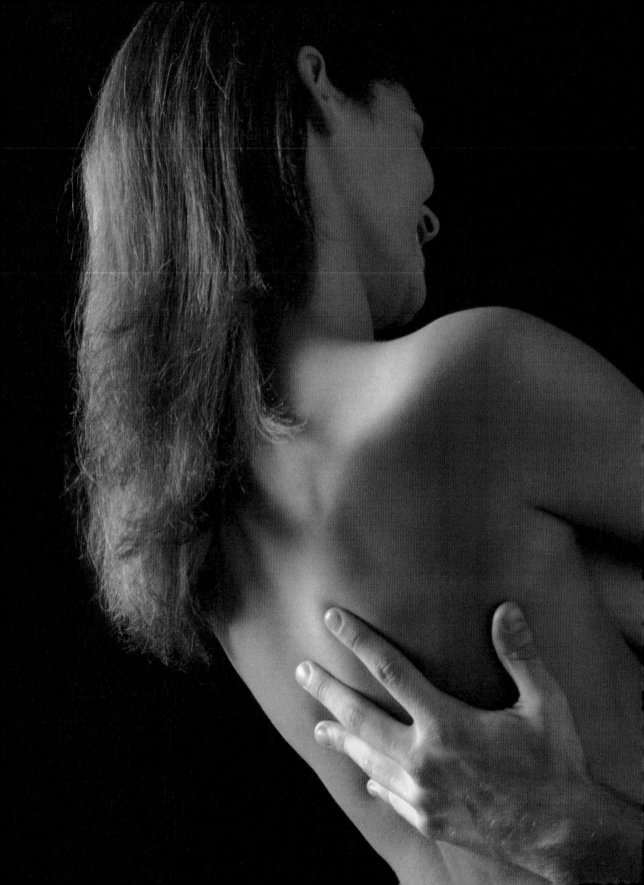

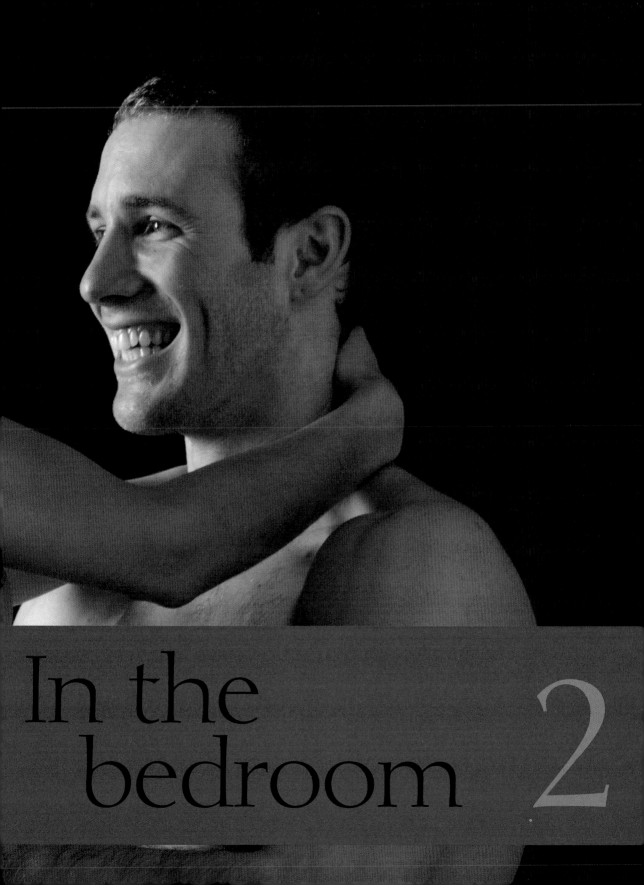

In the bedroom

2

Exploring your body

Many men and women have a tendency to believe that everybody has the same sexual response, but this is as incorrect as believing that all faces look the same. How you react to touch, how you experience it, and where you want to feel it, is unique to you: others' responses may be similar, but they are never the same.

Scalp and hair

The scalp is very sensitive to touch. It can be stimulated by direct fingertip massage or by running your fingers through the hair.

Although we are educated for many of the things we need as adults, most of us are taught virtually nothing that is relevant to our sex lives—other than the basics of reproduction. People in primitive societies often learned more than we do, especially if they lived in communal houses where they could actually see others making love. In many of those societies there were none of the taboos we place on sexual play for older children, and in some, the young people were paired with older ones who would initiate them into the mysteries of sex.

Yet today, school biology lessons focus first on nature, then on reproduction, and then, if you're lucky, on human reproduction—never on the physiology of pleasure. It would make a lot more sense if human physiology (including our sexual physiology) were studied first, and the birds and the bees made an optional extra.

How useful it would be to learn, for example, how hormones can influence us; that diet can affect us emotionally; that illnesses may create sexual side-effects; and that all these influences have a bearing on our love lives. These important details are often omitted from sex education.

If I were a schoolteacher, I would cover several subjects. How the body functions sexually; the physical changes experienced during arousal, orgasm, and resolution; how our bodies develop; how a healthy body may be enjoyed; and how to know when you are healthy are all vital areas of knowledge.

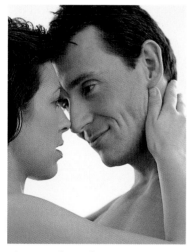

Ears and neck

These are among the most sensitive and erogenous parts of the body. Most people find that having their ears and neck stroked, nibbled, or licked is highly arousing, as are the sensations created by feeling a lover's hot breath in the ear.

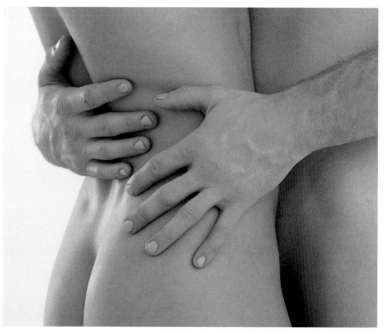

The waist

The waist is not often thought of as an erogenous zone, but there are many ways of touching it to create arousing feelings. It can be stroked, squeezed, and kissed for erotic effect, and some people like to have their navels touched and licked.

Erogenous zones

These and the following pages will provide you with this information about the human body and its responses. They contain the facts about male and female sexual response, plus two questionnaires. These are based on a routine invented by American sex therapists, William Hartman and Marilyn Fithian, that aims to give men and women detailed facts about their erogenous zones. The Sexual Body Questionnaire, for example, will provide you with knowledge of each other's skin reactions that you can put to good use when giving a sensual massage.

The value of answering these questionnaires together with your partner is that you can, in a way that provokes no feeling of criticism, let each other know what it is that you would really like. This is information you may have wanted to convey in the past but found difficult to bring out when actually in bed together.

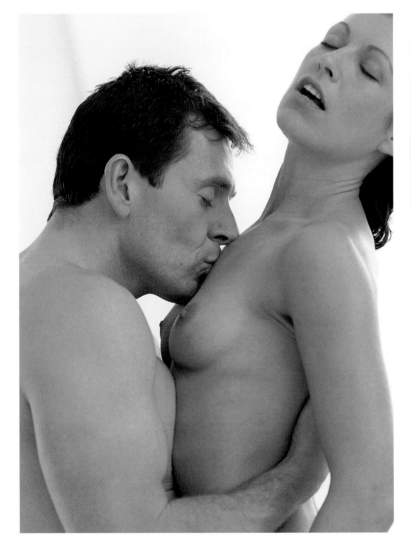

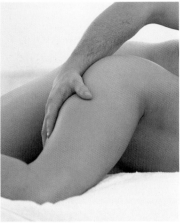

The thighs
The most sensitive parts of the thighs are the insides, and the closer the touch is to the groin, the more exquisite and arousing will be the sensations touching engenders.

The chest
Although not as sensitive as the breasts, the rest of the chest will respond pleasurably to sensual touch. Try light, teasing strokes and slow, lingering caresses.

SEXUAL BODY QUESTIONNAIRE

The goal of this questionnaire is to clarify your knowledge of each other's skin responses.

• If making love to yourself, where would you start?

• How long would you spend on this?

• Where does your partner habitually start when making love to you?

• How long does he/she spend on you?

• Which parts of your body make you feel sexy when they are touched? List them in order of preference, and think not just about the obvious areas, such as your genitals, breasts, and nipples, but also about the less obvious regions. These can include your scalp, hair, armpits, torso, waist, legs, ankles, and feet.

Breasts

A woman's breasts and nipples are obvious erogenous zones, but those of most men will also respond arousingly to manual and oral stimulation.

Gaining information

Although it has become easier to talk about sex, there is one aspect of lovemaking about which young people know even less now than they did 40 years ago. Thanks to the contraceptive pill, couples in new relationships tend to begin having intercourse without getting to know each other physically beforehand. The result: they miss out on gaining valuable, basic sexual information.

Breaking stereotypes

Many men incorrectly assume that women like their genitals touched immediately at the start of lovemaking, probably because this is an approach many men choose for themselves. Similarly, many women assume that men find it hard to be passive. Yet some men like the woman to make at least some of the moves first. By learning about each other's preferences, you can avoid thinking in terms of these old stereotypes.

Mutual pleasure

In finding out about each other's responses, you learn how to give each other sensual pleasure.

"The only good result of living in a world with HIV is that we have begun to learn methods of lovemaking other than intercourse."

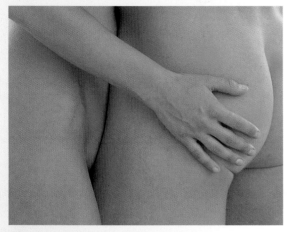

The buttocks

There are numerous ways of touching the buttocks to create arousing feelings, ranging from featherlight caresses to squeezing and even spanking.

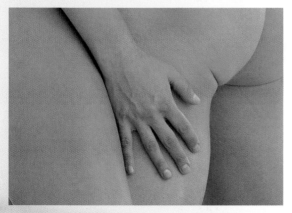

The backs of the legs

The fleshy back parts of the legs are generally more sensitive to touch than the fronts, and the hollows at the backs of the knees are especially so.

TOUCH INTENSITY QUESTIONNAIRE

This questionnaire, like the Sexual Body Questionnaire on page 47, is one you can work through with your partner. It is intended to give each of you an insight into how the other likes to be touched during foreplay and intercourse.

- Do you like:
  rough touch
  soft touch
  firm touch
  light touch
- Do you prefer touch to be:
  fast
  slow
- In lovemaking, is it more exciting if:
  you take the initiative
  your lover takes the initiative
  everything happens spontaneously

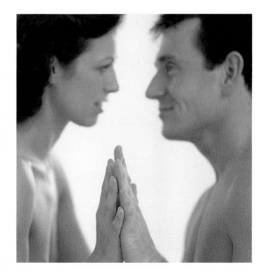

A man's sensuality

To get an idea of your partner's erogenous zones, begin by looking at the order in which he rated the parts of his body in our Sexual Body Questionnaire (*see page 47*). Then give him the Sensitivity Test, which will help you to visualize the pattern of his erotic responses.

With your partner lying unclothed, perform the Sensitivity Test by exploring and stroking the preferred areas of his body with your fingertips. As you do so, ask your partner to rate your strokes on a scale of plus three to minus three. For example, if something feels wonderful, he might rate this as plus three on the scale; if there is little sensation, as either plus one or zero; or if it feels unpleasant or painful, he could use the minus ratings. In this way

Stroking action

When you are performing the Sensitivity Test, use light but firm pressure and make short, circular strokes with your forefinger and middle finger.

you can build up a detailed mental image of what feels good to him and what does not.

Teaching increased response

It is possible to build up erotic sensation with rhythmic stimulation once your partner feels you have got the touch right, but this is just a fact-finding mission: there is no orgasmic end in mind. Your job is to gain information, and his is to offer it. Together, you are working out the best possible combination of your ability to touch and his ability to appreciate it.

The penis and testicles

The American sex researchers Masters and Johnson found that, instead of remaining at one expanded size, there are degrees of expansion for the penis during sexual arousal. If penile stimulation is prolonged, apparently well-established erections continue to expand. Although this expansion was demonstrated using oral or manual methods of stimulation, Masters and Johnson hypothesize that there is every reason to think the same expansion would continue during prolonged intercourse.

The testicles begin to expand in diameter late in the arousal phase. The only times when testicular expansion was not demonstrated in the Masters and Johnson survey was when men ejaculated very rapidly after onset of stimulation. If sexual excitement is kept high for a long time without the release of ejaculation, then most men experience a severe ache in the testicles. This can be quickly relieved by ejaculation.

The nipples

In 1979, Masters and Johnson published a valuable study of homosexual behavior. One of its findings was that homosexual men usually pay much more attention to their partners' nipples at the beginning of foreplay than do heterosexuals, and they stimulate them both manually and orally.

Heterosexual couples can learn a great deal from this. Part of what makes any area of the body feel good when touched is a sense of comfort and an acceptance of that touch. Even if a man's nipples have never possessed much sensation before, it may be possible, through some good experience and practice, for him to respond erotically.

WARM TOUCH

Just as you do before giving a massage, ensure that your hands are comfortably warm before you begin your exploration of your partner's skin.

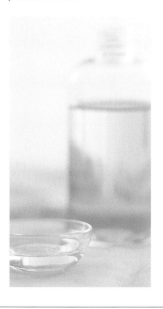

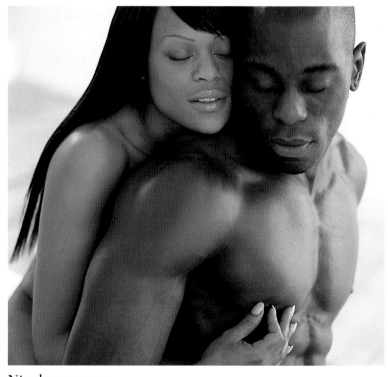

Nipple response

If he tells you he would like to feel more in his nipples, ask him to take your hands and hold them over his nipples, demonstrating the movements and pressures that feel good.

Expand your repertoire

Don't be afraid to learn from others, be they heterosexual or homosexual. Research shows gay couples spend a long time on sensual caressing.

Male sexual response

In general, men are more quickly and easily aroused than women, but after orgasm they usually have to wait much longer before they are able to have intercourse again. The most obvious sign of male arousal is erection of the penis, but other physical changes also take place.

Messages of sexual arousal from the brain or the spinal cord can travel to the genitals within 10 to 30 seconds of stimulation. With men, the principal effect of this is erection of the penis, which is caused by the intricate network of vessels within its spongelike erectile tissues filling with blood.

In addition to penile erection, the testes are pulled up toward the body and the wall of the scrotum gets thicker and tighter. If stimulation is prolonged or intensified, the testes are pulled up farther and increase in size. As sexual excitement increases, blood pressure rises, and heart rate and skin temperature increase. The pupils dilate, and the nipples may become erect.

Muscle tension in men also increases during arousal. Breathing becomes almost hyperventilation and many men experience a "sex flush," a kind of reddish rash under the skin of the head and chest. After orgasm, these changes disappear very rapidly, and for a varying length of time (known as the refractory period), few men can be stimulated once more to climax.

Orgasm

Alfred Kinsey described the male orgasm as "an explosive discharge of neuromuscular tension" during which "the individual suddenly becomes tense, momentarily maintains a high level of tension, rises to a new peak of maximum tension—and then abruptly

Varied sensations

There are many different ways of experiencing orgasm—it can be felt across the entire body, or sometimes it is a purely genital sensation.

Sex flush

During the most intense phase of sexual arousal, about 25 percent of men show a reddening below the skin of the head and chest.

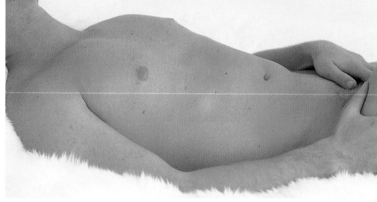

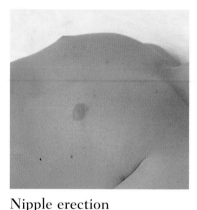

Nipple erection

Up to 60 percent of men experience nipple erection when they become sexually aroused, but the remaining 40 percent or so show no visible signs of erection.

"Men recognize that orgasm is imminent when they reach what's known as the 'point of no return'—a sense of inevitable ejaculation."

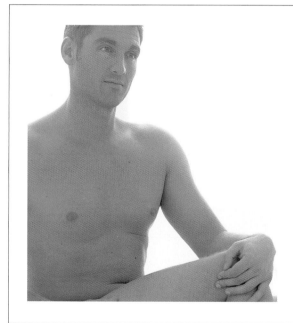

THE MALE RESPONSE CYCLE

In the latest definition of the sexual response cycle, its first three stages are desire, arousal, and orgasm. Desire is a hard-to-quantify emotion, which some say is an attitude of mind and others the product of hormone activity, and it often blends with the next stage, arousal. Some men become aroused with little or no physical stimulation, but others may need a great deal. As stimulation continues, by hand or during the thrusting of intercourse, a man's arousal and excitement intensify and lead to orgasm and ejaculation. Excitement and erection then subside and he enters the refractory phase, in which his body slowly returns to normal. During this period, some men may be able to have another erection, but usually not another ejaculation.

and instantaneously releases all tensions and plunges in a series of muscular spasms, or convulsions, through which he returns to a normal or even subnormal physiologic state."

Men recognize that orgasm is imminent when they reach what's known as the "point of no return"—a sense of inevitable ejaculation. The semen is pumped out through the urethra by short bursts of intense muscular contraction. Interestingly, the rhythmic muscular contractions of the penis during ejaculation occur at the same rate as do the contractions of the vagina during female climax (*see page 66*).

The amount of semen ejaculated varies considerably and can be anything between one and six milliliters in volume, that is, up to about a teaspoonful. If there is repeated ejaculation over a short period, the amount of semen produced each time gradually diminishes. On the other hand, if a long time has passed since the previous ejaculation, the amount produced is likely to be relatively large.

Orgasm can lead to an altered state of consciousness. In most men and women, this means a sense of being "on a different level" of the brain, rather than of actually losing consciousness.

Muscle tension and heartbeat

During sexual arousal, the muscles become increasingly tense, the heart rate increases, and there is a slight rise in blood pressure. These changes intensify until after orgasm, when the body reverts to normal.

Male multiple orgasms

A few men are capable of multiple orgasm (more than one orgasm in a session). American sex researchers Hartman and Fithian discovered that it may not be linked with ejaculation, and that men might be able to experience climaxes without ejaculation.

All-around benefits

Not all men are able to have a multiple orgasm, but even if you are unable to become multiorgasmic, these exercises will increase your genital fitness and give you greater ejaculatory control.

The men studied by Hartman and Fithian in their research seem to have achieved multiple orgasms by tensing their thigh muscles and squeezing their pelvic floor or PC (pubococcygeal) muscles. In doing so, they would have blocked off their ejaculations by closing their urethral tubes with muscle action. This is like an internal version of the squeeze technique of ejaculation control (*see page 117*). But because the male climax is so associated with ejaculation, nobody knows, even in the laboratory, if these multiorgasmic males were actually climaxing or were simply experiencing peaks of excitement. Whatever it was that they were doing, however, they were clearly undergoing an intense sexual experience.

Get training!

According to Nick Konnoff, a star subject of Hartman and Fithian's laboratory tests, there is a training routine to help you achieve multiple orgasm. The routine consists of four sets of simple exercises (*see right*) which lead to longer-lasting sexual arousal and more intense climaxes. You may find that you need more sex as a result of doing the exercises.

TRAINING FOR MULTIPLE ORGASM

Flexing the PC muscles
Develop your PC and inner groin muscles by waving your penis around by using these muscles alone, or try to lift a washcloth on your erect penis. Do this at least twice a day.

Testicle control
The testicles rise automatically before climax. Learning to raise them may make ejaculation easier; lowering them may delay it. Stand with feet apart and pull your testicle muscles up toward your abdomen. Increase repetitions daily.

Erection maintenance
Give yourself an erection and continue it for as long as possible by both manual and emotional stimulation. Start by trying for a minute a day for the first week and build up from there.

Myotonic exercise
Climax is triggered by pelvic tension called *myotonia*. To build this up, alternately flex and relax your legs and lower abdomen. Aim to do this for five minutes, but stop if you begin to cramp.

A woman's sensuality

The peaks of a woman's sexual sensation correspond to those of a man, but certain areas of the body will feel more sensitive. Use the Sensitivity Test (*see page 50*) to find out which areas they are.

To help your partner increase her response to sexual stimulation, build up a variety of sensation on the less obviously erotic places, such as the neck and the shoulders, and on the torso at the sides of the breast. By stimulating these areas with stroking, light scratching, gentle biting, and tongue bathing, and then proceeding, believe it or not, to the feet, you will induce a highly charged state of sexual desire in your partner's body. Then, and only then, you can touch her genitals to find out how much she feels and where.

The breasts

In their 1979 study of homosexual sexual response, Masters and Johnson found that lesbian women, when making love, began by holding, kissing, and caressing each

Genital stimulation

Leave her genitals until last. Your goal should be to find out more about her response to stimulation of her labia, vagina, and clitoris, and not, at this point, to try bringing her to orgasm.

other's whole body for much longer than heterosexual couples do. When the lesbian couples finally turned to specific parts of the body, the breasts received much more attention, and for far longer, than was typical in heterosexual lovemaking.

The whole breast was caressed, both manually and orally, with special concentration on the nipples. Approximately equal amounts of time were taken on each breast, and sometimes as much as 10 minutes was spent on breast caressing before turning to the genitals. The woman being stimulated always produced copious vaginal secretions at this time, and on two separate occasions one of the study subjects actually climaxed strongly during breast play alone, before her genitals had been touched.

Interestingly, the women in Masters and Johnson's study of heterosexual couples reported that their breasts were not a particularly erogenous zone to them. There are lessons to be learned from this, probably the most important being that even if heterosexual women don't experience much breast sensation, they have the potential for it. Experimenting with breast massage is one way of awakening a woman's erotic breast sensation.

"Some women experience a height of sensuality through fabulous body stimulation."

The torso

The sides of the torso can be surprisingly responsive to touch, especially to light, brushing, fingertip strokes and to licking and gentle nibbling.

The labia and clitoris

The external female genitalia are referred to collectively as the vulva. This consists of the outer labia (vaginal lips); the inner labia; the clitoris, which is usually covered by the mons pubis or pubic mound (the fleshy pad above the genitals, clothed in pubic hair); and the entrance to the vagina. Inside this entrance, near the top, is the urinary opening.

The outer and inner labia can vary greatly in size. Some women have small, fleshy outer labia and long, hanging inner labia. Others possess highly developed outer labia, and very small inner labia that look very much like a fringe around the vaginal entrance. And there are many dozens of styles in between.

The outer lips are often hairy on the outside but, when pulled open, show a paler shade on the inside. The inner lips may also be a paler color on the inside than on the outside. The colors deepen with age. It is normal for one labium to hang lower than the other and for one side of the clitoral hood to fall lower than the other. It is also normal for some women to possess extremely hairy genitals and for others to have virtually no pubic hair. There is great variation in genital appearance from one woman to another.

A man can probably maximize his partner's response to clitoral stimulation by following a similar procedure to that employed by the lesbian women in Masters and Johnson's studies. These women almost always caressed each other's labia, mons pubis, inner thighs, and vaginal entrance before touching the clitoris. And when clitoral stimulation had begun, even though the head of the clitoris may have been stroked initially, the focus of the stimulation usually became the clitoral shaft.

The couples used two main kinds of sex play. The first was a "teasing cycle," in which one partner stimulated the other to the point of orgasm and then allowed her arousal to subside before stimulating her further. In the second, one partner stimulated the other with more continuity and increasing intensity until she climaxed. Lesbians rarely used their fingers to penetrate each other's vagina. This happened quite regularly among the heterosexual couples, however, but the women involved derived little pleasure from it.

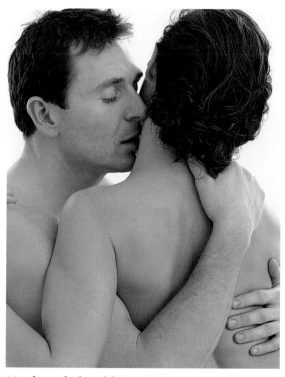

Neck and shoulders

To begin exploring your partner's responses to stimulation, gently kiss her lips and then work your way slowly down her neck and across each of her shoulders.

Female sexual response

Although a woman's genitals are mostly hidden within her body, their external parts—principally the clitoris, the inner and outer labia, and the opening to the vagina—are extremely sensitive to touch. Despite this sensitivity, women are generally not as quickly aroused as men, but after orgasm it takes longer for their arousal to subside.

The first sign of female arousal is vaginal lubrication. The vagina lengthens and distends, and the vaginal walls change to a darker color because of engorgement with blood. This engorgement, which in men is responsible for filling and elevating the penis, in women fills the labia and the clitoral shaft.

The breasts swell, the nipples become erect, and the uterus and cervix begin to move upward. Heart rate and blood pressure increase, while a sex flush can appear on the skin.

As excitement grows, many muscles become tense. Other reactions include jerking of limbs, trembling, and the thrusting of genitals. During acute excitement, the outer third of the vagina (the orgasmic platform) closes a little due to the increased blood supply. The engorged inner labia change color dramatically to a brighter or deeper red.

When the woman has entered the pre-orgasm, *plateau phase*, her uterus also engorges and continues to grow, rising farther up in the pelvis. This creates *tenting*, caused when this elevation lifts the cervix and leaves a space at the far end of the vagina. The walls of the vagina also exude a secretion.

At this stage, the clitoris retracts into the swollen pubis and the tissues around the nipples swell with fluid, enlarging the areolae and making the nipple erection disappear. Heart rate and blood pressure continue to increase.

Muscular tension

General tension of the muscles and limbs increases with increasing arousal, and it often culminates, at orgasm, in powerful, involuntary muscular spasms.

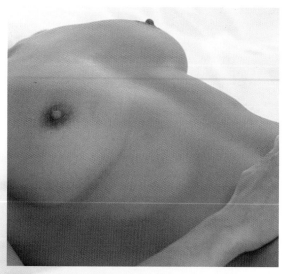

Orgasm

Climax begins with muscular contractions, originating in the orgasmic platform, which contracts rhythmically as sexual tension is released. Masters and Johnson found that these orgasmic contractions usually occurred from three to 15 times and at 0.8-second intervals, decreasing in frequency and intensity after the first few. This pattern of contractions is the same as that of the penis during a man's ejaculation. Sometimes, a woman's uterus and anus also contract simultaneously and powerfully during orgasm.

Nipple erection

Nipple erection begins in the excitement phase and peaks at orgasm, but may be hidden by enlargement of the breasts and areolae during intense excitement.

Sex flush

In most women, a sex flush appears during the excitement phase of the response cycle, intensifies with increase arousal, and is at its most intense during orgasm.

At the moment of orgasm, breathing is at least three times as fast as it would be normally, the heartbeat more than double its usual rate, and the blood pressure is increased by one-third. Most of the body muscles are tense.

After orgasm comes the *resolution phase*. During this phase, in some women the body returns to its previously unstimulated state, with the clitoris returning to its normal size and position, the vagina returning to its normal size, and the uterus and cervix dropping back to their normal position. In other women, however, the body merely drops back into the excitement stage before going on to further orgasms (provided that stimulation continues).

Status orgasmus

There is also a particular orgasmic response, noted by Masters and Johnson, which they call *status orgasmus*. In this, a few women are able to have a rapidly recurrent set of orgasms with no intermittent resting phase (*see page 69*). Women who experience this response may be able to identify different peaks, or they may simply feel that they are going through an intensely long climax, with no identifiable separate peaks.

"According to Dr. Helen Singer Kaplan, each of the three phases—desire, arousal, and orgasm—can be experienced separately as well as in a sequence."

THE FEMALE RESPONSE CYCLE

A woman's sexual response cycle, like that of a man (*see page 56*), begins with desire. Arousal and excitement are the next stages, and while some women are ready for orgasm almost immediately, others need up to 45 minutes of stimulation before orgasm is possible.

The arousal phase is followed by orgasm, in which orgasmic contractions occur in a similar way to those of the man. The majority of women then experience a loss of sexual and muscular tension after orgasm.

But there is a major difference here between male and female sexual response in that a minority of women, unlike men, can remain highly aroused and capable of further orgasms.

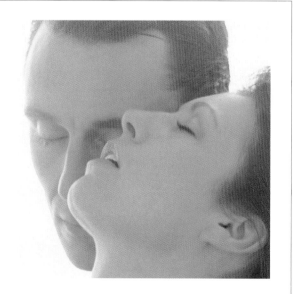

Female multiple orgasms

Women have turned out to possess a sexual advantage over men: a sizeable minority can experience multiple orgasms. For some, all it takes is continued stimulation after the first climax. Sadly, only a very few men can manage this.

Arousal

A high level of sexual arousal before your initial climax, and continuing stimulation after it, can help you to have multiple orgasms. Telling each other sexual fantasies will increase your arousal.

Multiple orgasm can be experienced in a number of different ways, but it usually consists of a series of separate orgasms occurring within a short time, sometimes with only a few seconds between them, sometimes with longer intervals. Some women experience multiple orgasm as a series of gentle peaks that feel connected, while others have one strong climax after another, each one seeming to run into the next.

To be able to achieve multiple orgasm, a woman needs continuing stimulation after her initial climax. Her partner must be able to control his ejaculation so that he can keep thrusting, or else provide her with manual stimulation after he himself has climaxed and withdrawn. The chances of having multiple orgasms are also increased if the woman is given a high level of sexual stimulation before intercourse begins.

Orgasmic capability

Not all women are capable of multiple orgasms, and not all women want them. Many women find satisfaction from one good orgasm, and others feel too sensitive for continuing stimulation after one orgasm.

No one yet knows why some women, but not others, should be able to have multiple orgasms, but one theory has it that the ability is due to high levels of free-ranging testosterone within the body. Our hormone levels are either random or may be inherited in the same way as other physical characteristics. A woman's state of health is also known to affect her hormone balance, as do medications such as the contraceptive pill.

Women who are more easily aroused can usually experience multiple orgasm during intercourse. Some women discover, in their late 20s or early 30s, that they can learn how to have more than one climax when stimulating themselves or while being masturbated. Women are at their sexual peak in their early 30s, so maybe this is reflecting high testosterone levels. But it can also reflect a better knowledge of one's own sexual response and greater self-confidence. Encouragingly, studies have shown that women in their 30s are much more likely than younger women to be capable of having multiple orgasms.

If you have not experienced multiple orgasms but want to discover if you are capable of being multiorgasmic, you might like to try a simple training program (*see below*). Success cannot be guaranteed, alas, but you can enjoy trying.

TRAINING FOR MULTIPLE ORGASM

Increase arousal

Useful techniques for increasing your level of sexual arousal include enjoying a dramatic sexual fantasy, watching a sexy movie, and delaying orgasm. Instead of going for orgasm at the first possible opportunity, wait. Put it off, again and again, until you reach an extreme pitch of arousal (some women find this easier and less tiring to do if they use a vibrator instead of their fingers).

Continue stimulation

When you reach climax, continue with the stimulation. You may find that your orgasm goes on for much longer than you would have expected.

Think positively

If you accept, on first climax, that you're finished for the day, then you're likely to be just that. Try keeping your mind full of erotic thoughts.

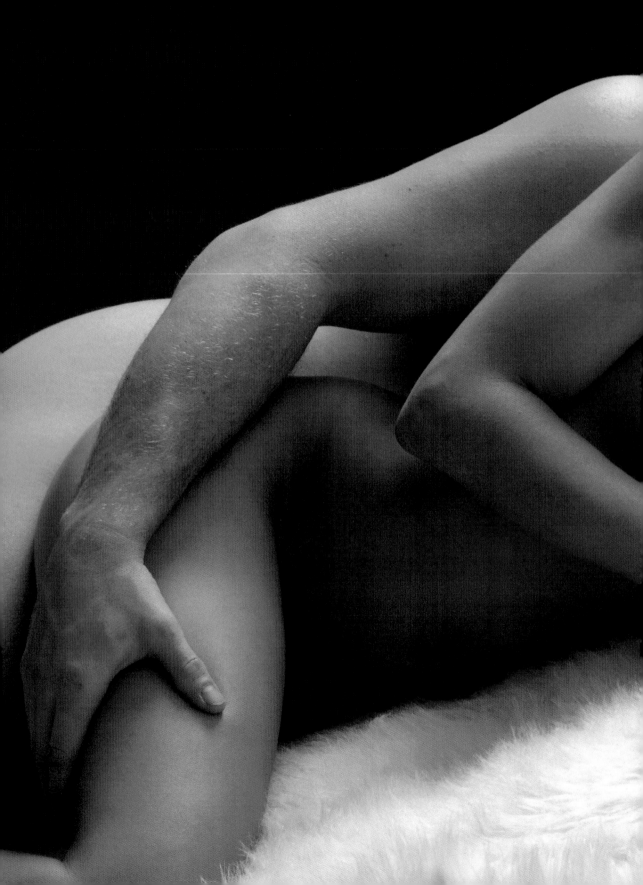

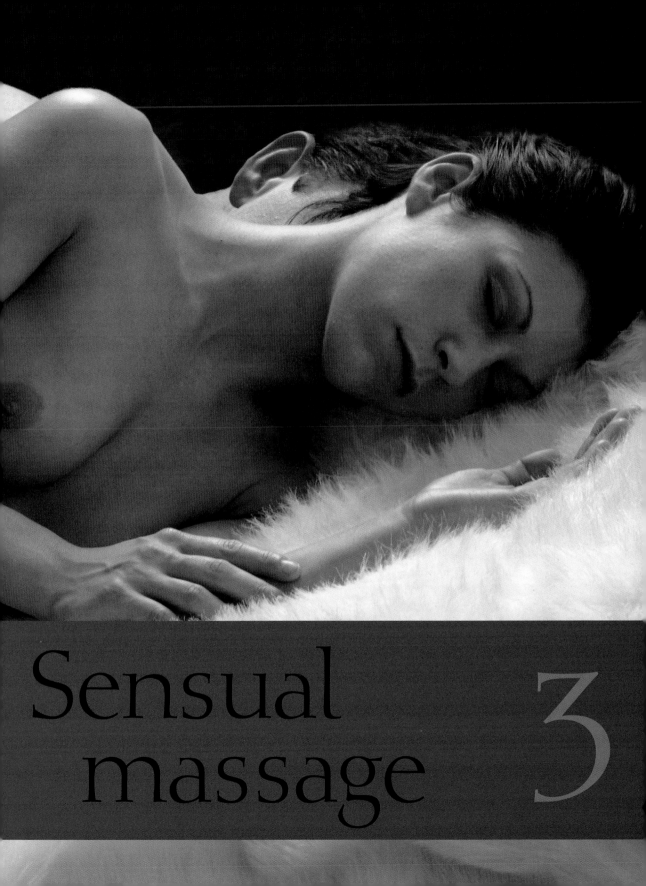

Sensual massage

3

The joy of massage

Most of us believe that feeling sensual is allowable only within the framework of lovemaking, preferably with a committed partner. Yet there is a wealth of wonderful sensation at our fingertips which can be given to others or to ourselves.

Accepting that we all deserve such pleasure, and that there is nothing wrong or abnormal about it, opens us up to great delights. The starting point for this comes in the shape of whole-body sensual massage. You don't have to do this with a committed partner for it to be sensational, but of course it feels especially good when you offer your tantalizing touch to the one you love.

On the following pages you will find the strokes that make up a whole-body massage. Before we discuss them, spare a little time to consider some important details. These are details that make the difference between a matter-of-fact present of touch and a mysterious, overwhelming, spiritual gift. That's a strong promise, but massage can offer stimulation for the brain as well as for the body.

Patterns

As you get to know which strokes you feel most comfortable with giving, you will understand that it makes sense to carry out strokes in certain patterns. For example, working your way up one side of the body and then down the other is a pattern. And alternating grand, sweeping strokes with little, detailed strokes is another pattern. Remember to include as much of the body as possible so that no part feels left out.

Timing

Massage can be tiring, so don't overdo it on the first occasions. I always feel so overwhelmed by a good back massage that I don't instantly long for my front to get attention, but many people feel cheated if the front is ignored. If both front and back massage is required, cut down on the number of strokes for each so that what you do deliver is done with freshness and energy.

Don't expect to use every single one of the strokes described on the following pages. To

Agreement

Before you begin, you should both agree exactly what is going to happen during the session, and change your plan only by mutual consent.

TEN GOLDEN RULES

- Respect your partner's requests
- Honor any agreement you make in advance of the session, for example, that intercourse is not on the agenda
- Keep your massage movements slow
- Be aware of the sensations you receive when giving a massage
- Try to tune in to your partner's reaction to your massage gift
- Never foist a massage on someone who says he or she does not want it
- Make a point of gently asking your partner for feedback
- When it's your turn to be massaged, remember to give your partner plenty of tactful feedback
- Ensure that you have privacy
- Make sure that the room, your hands, and the massage oil are warm

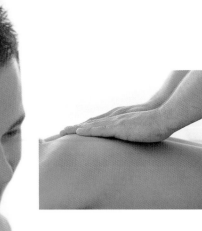

Sweeping strokes

When you are massaging relatively large areas of the body, such as the back, use long, sensuous, sweeping strokes and try to keep the sensations your partner feels as smooth and continuous as possible.

Comfort

A massage should be unhurried and performed in warm, comfortable surroundings. The massage surface should be firm and covered in soft sheets or towels. Clothes, if worn, should be soft, loose-fitting, and comfortable.

conserve your energy, try a few different ones on every occasion; this will also help you to learn which are the most effective. If asking for feedback proves brutally intrusive, remember to check with your partner afterward for details of how he or she enjoyed the massage.

One of the keys to making a massage truly heavenly is to feel it yourself as a sensual experience. Close your eyes, feel the sensation on your hands, and alter your touch so that it pleases you as well as your partner.

Setting the scene

A cluttered room is not going to have the same visual impact on the would-be sensualist as a room with exotic colors and low lighting. Clean towels, sheets, and coverings are essential. And if oil spills are likely, protect the massage surface by covering it with something washable, such as a towel.

Some people like soft and tasteful music playing in the background during a massage session. But if you don't have a machine that will repeat the tape or CD, position the player near you so that you can easily put on something new; if music is part of the spell you are creating, it can be distracting if it suddenly stops. In that case, it would be better to have no music at all.

The smell of incense is an erotic addition to the ambience of the massage scene. You could use burning joss sticks or warm, sweet-smelling oil in a candle-fired burner. The massage oil itself should also smell exotic. Many herbalists and health stores stock oils suitable for massage, and if you want a stronger smell, you can always add a perfume to these oils.

Detailed strokes
The strokes you use on the smaller, more complicated parts of the body, such as the shoulders, hands, and feet, should be short but decisive. Avoid massaging areas where the bone is close to the skin.

Back massage

Many of these strokes can be used on the front of the body (*see pages 84–89*) as well as on the back, but the back is the easiest part of the anatomy to begin with. It offers you a relatively large area on which to work, and because it is less sensitive than the front, it is a good part of the body on which to discover how to adjust the pressure of your strokes.

For a back massage, your partner lies face down. You kneel or sit alongside, and work up from the buttocks to the shoulders. Begin by coating your partner's back with warm massage oil, using sweeping, flowing strokes and spreading it generously over his or her skin.

When you start on the massage itself, don't forget the golden rule: take it slowly. Being lingered over is far more sensual than being rushed at like an old washboard, so take your time over it. And, as a general principle, if either of you feels that things have gone ahead too far, too fast, go back a stage so that you are both able to feel secure again.

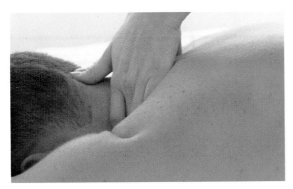

Hairline circling

After circling up the back, massage from the tops of the arms across the shoulders to the neck and let your thumbs circle into the hairline.

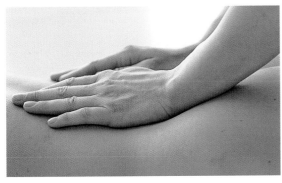

The glide

Place both hands flat on the buttocks, then lean forward and let your weight push your hands up your partner's body. Repeat once.

Circling

This is the first and most basic stroke, and it can also be used as a link between other strokes. Place both hands, palms downward, on the shoulders and move them firmly in opposing circles. Work out and away from the spine, progressing down the back and over the buttocks. Then work back up to the shoulders and repeat twice.

TIPS FOR A SENSUAL BACK MASSAGE

- Pressure is the secret of turning a routine massage into a sensual experience. A strong massage feels thorough and "medical," a lighter one pleasurable and sensual, and a fingertip massage arousing and erotic.
- Timing is also important: if you give someone a fingertip massage without preceding it with a firmer one, your touch can be felt as irritating or even tickling.

- The skin needs to be prepared for its arousal, which may be why, when making love, time spent snuggling, stroking, and rubbing bodies together is such an important precursor to more intimate foreplay.
- Feedback from your partner will tell you which strokes feel good and which are less successful. Create a mental "relief map" of your partner's erogenous zones (see page 50).

Lower spine massage

Lean heavily on your hands and let your weight force them slowly apart, so that they slip down the sides of the body to the ground or bed. Just before your hands reach the ground or bed, repeat the stroke, starting nearer the base of the spine. Repeat as many times as your partner wants.

ADDING MORE

To apply more oil, keep the back of one hand resting on your partner's skin, cup it, and pour a little oil into it.

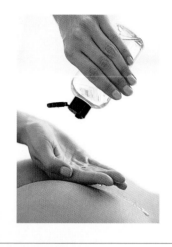

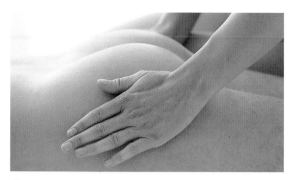

Cross-currents

This is a variation of circling. Use the palms of your hands, moving them close together in opposing circles, and work over the fleshy areas of the back and the buttocks.

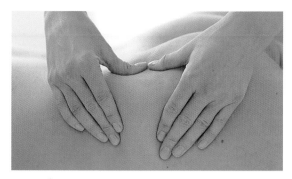

Kneading

Kneading is good for the hips, the buttocks, and fleshy areas of the back. Using the thumbs and forefingers of both hands, rhythmically squeeze and release the skin.

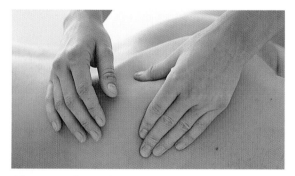

Alternate kneading

In this variation of the basic kneading stroke, you gently squeeze your partner's flesh with one hand at a time instead of using both hands simultaneously.

Thumbing

Using both thumbs, make short, rapid, alternate strokes on the lower back. You can either move your thumbs in circular strokes or simply push them upward. Beginning on your partner's buttocks and gradually moving up to the waist, work your way up one side of the back and then up the other.

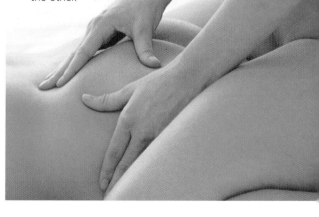

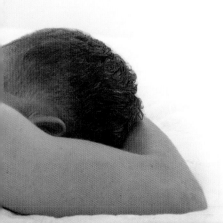

THE CATERPILLAR

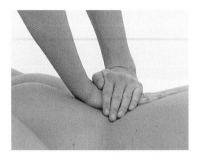 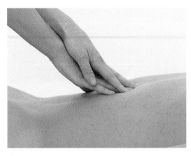 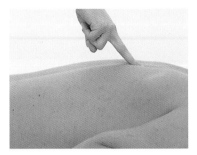

1 Sit at your partner's side and place your left hand on the base of the spine, pointing to the head. Place your right hand on top of your left.

2 Slowly glide forward on the palm and back on the fingers, pushing down with the right hand; work your way caterpillar-like up the spine.

3 At the top, take your right hand away. Press the first two fingers of your left hand slowly down each side of the spine. Repeat the strokes twice.

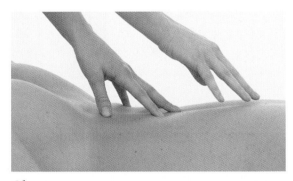

Stop-start clawing
Work your middle and forefingers along the "grooves" on each side of the spine, working all the way down.

Clawing
With only your fingertips resting on the skin, pull down firmly hand over hand along one side of the body and then the other.

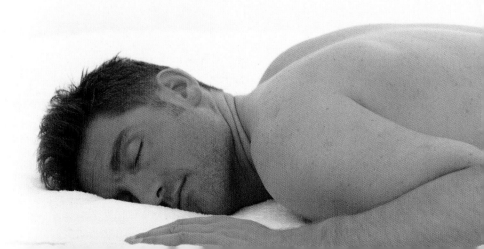

"If you are being massaged, relax your upper-body muscles so that the effect of the massage is not diminished by your muscular tension."

Easing the lower spine

The base of the spine takes the constant pressure of keeping the body upright all day. This soothing lower spine massage is intended to relieve some of the tension caused by that pressure. To begin the massage, kneel astride your partner and place a hand on each side of the spine, just below the waist, with your fingers pointing sideways.

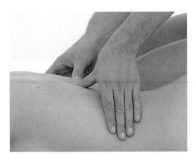

Spinal tap

Press your thumbs into the indentations on either side of your partner's spine, and draw them slowly down until you reach the base. Repeat.

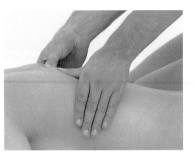

The thumb slide

In this reverse spinal tap, push your thumbs firmly up on either side of the spine, from the base to the hairline. Repeat, varying the pressure.

The hip lift

Glide your hands down the body from the shoulders to the buttocks, then slip your hands under the hips and draw them up the underside of the body to lift it slightly.
Repeat once.

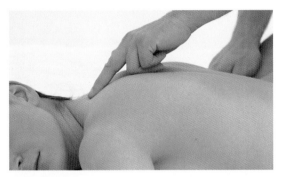

One hand only

Press on the spine just below the neck with your forefinger and middle finger, then slowly pull them down the spine, keeping the pressure even. Repeat.

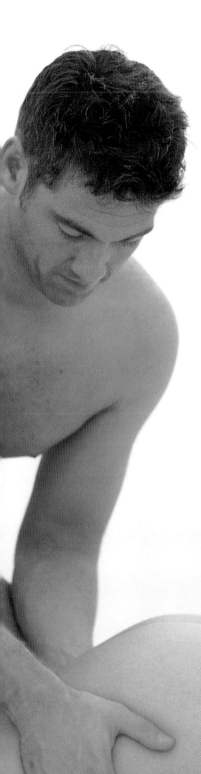

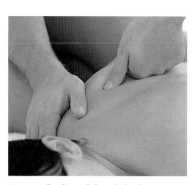

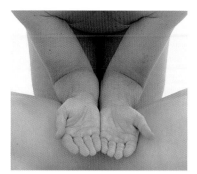

Raised shoulder blade

This is a fairly difficult stroke, so don't panic if you find it hard to carry out. The first stage is to fold one of your partner's arms across the back, then slip your arm under the forearm until the elbow is resting in the crook of your arm. Now lever up your arm slightly, and you will see your partner's shoulder blade lift.

The second stage of this stroke is to press your thumb into the space below the shoulder blade, then draw it out to the armpit. Do this three or four times, then repeat on the other side.

Finishing off

Kneeling at your partner's side, place the backs of your forearms close together across the center of his or her body. Then very slowly spread your arms apart and turn them slightly inward.

By the time your arms have reached the neck and buttocks, the fronts of your forearms should be in contact with your partner's body. When your arms meet the neck and buttocks, lift them off and repeat the stroke. On the third repetition, slow the movement down and, when you finish, lift your arms off as gently as possible and sit quietly.

Front massage

In addition to the strokes shown here, many of those used in back massage (*see pages 76–83*) can also be used in front massage. If you are following up a back massage with a front massage, help your partner to turn over slowly. Rolling over, rather than sitting up suddenly, is the gentlest method.

Begin by coating your partner with massage oil. If your partner is male and has a hairy chest, apply extra oil to it so that your fingers don't catch. If your partner is female, remember to include her breasts in the massage (*see page 90*).

In back massage, circling is the basic stroke and the one that is used to link other strokes. In front massage, the slide takes its place and is the best stroke with which to begin the massage. When using the slide, kneel at your partner's head and place your hands, palms down, on the chest, with the heels of your hands next to the armpits. Then lean forward and slide your hands down over your partner's body.

Next, give your partner a shoulder lift and head lift, and caress his or her head. Then work on the chest (*see pages 86–87*), using fairy rings on the upper chest and cupping strokes on the breasts.

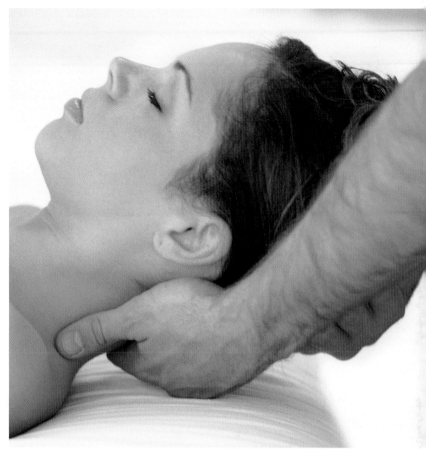

Caressing the head

Keeping your partner's head supported, repeatedly draw each alternate hands from the nape of the neck to the crown.

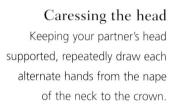

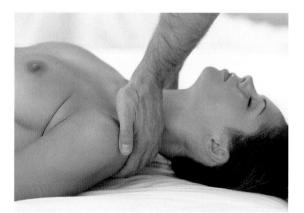

The shoulder lift

Slip your hands underneath your partner's shoulders, then firmly draw them up and out, lifting the shoulders slightly as you do so.

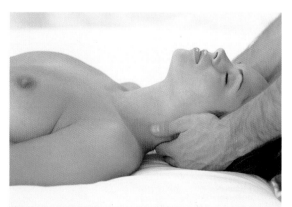

The head lift

A variation on the shoulder lift is to pull your hands along the underside of the head, with your fingers against the back of the neck.

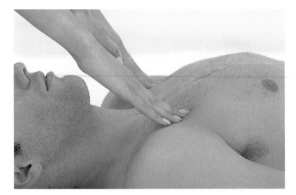

The slide

Lean forward and let your weight carry your hands down the body until you can reach no farther; repeat two times. If your partner is female, reduce the pressure when your fingers begin to slip over her breasts.

Fairy rings

Using the fingertips of both hands and starting at the collar bones, make tiny circles over the whole of the upper chest except the breasts.

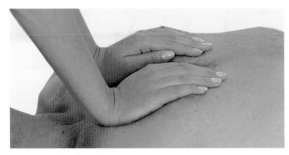

Cupping the breasts

Using cupped hands, gently rotate the breasts as fully as possible, moving them clockwise, counterclockwise, and in opposite directions.

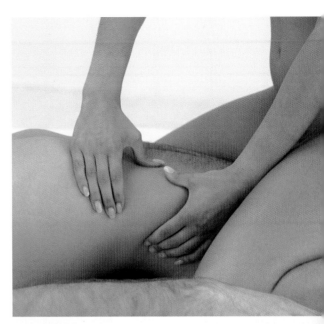

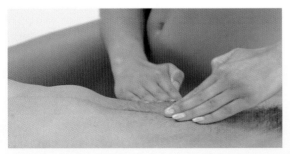

Using both hands

Vary the belly circling strokes by using your other hand as well. Make semicircles with it from hip to hip, moving in the same direction as the first hand and lifting off every time that hand comes around. A further variation is to continue your clockwise circles with one hand, only this time twist the hand itself for part of its run so that you are then massaging with the back of the hand.

Kneading

This is done on the front of the body in the same way as it is on the back (see page 79), focusing on the fleshy areas around the waist and the hips. As before, you can use both hands either simultaneously or alternately, and once you've covered all the suitably fleshy areas, vary the sensation by deep circling with the tips of the fingers.

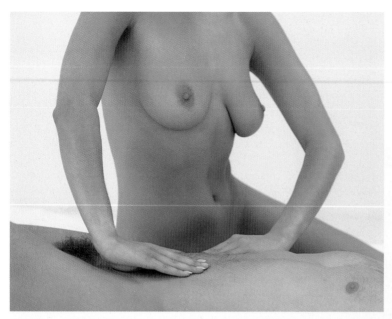

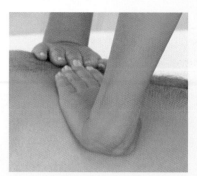

The abdominal twist

To vary the abdominal slide, twist your hands so that their heels face outward and the fingertips meet at your partner's middle. Gently sweep these apart below the rib cage so that your fingertips trace the bottom ribs.

Circling the belly

It is sensible to leave the belly massage strokes until last, because by this stage in the session your partner's body will have gotten used to being touched and ticklishness is less likely. Should ticklishness be a problem, however, you can usually overcome it by using a firm touch. Massage in a clockwise direction (the direction in which the colon runs), and use the palm of one hand to make full circles along the outer rim of the belly.

The abdominal slide

In this stroke, you slide your hands firmly but gently up your partner's abdomen from groin to ribs. Before you start, straddle comfortably across your partner's thighs. Place both palms on your partner's lower abdomen, with your fingers pointing toward the head. Then push your hands (not by leaning on them, because your weight would be too much) slowly up the abdomen until your fingertips meet the rib cage. Repeat as desired.

FIRST AND SECOND SPINAL TAPS

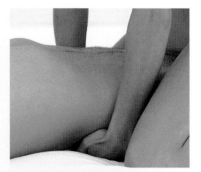 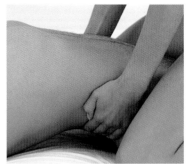

1 Slip your hands underneath each side of your partner's waist and move your fingertips so that they are positioned on each side of the spine. Keeping the backs of your hands against the floor, press up with your fingertips firmly enough to lift your partner just a little bit. Hold the position for a count of 20 and then let him or her down slowly.

2 Put your hands beneath your partner and lace your fingers tightly together under the spine. Then pull up and toward you, so that your partner is lifted slightly and then settles gently back.

Note This is an excellent move with which to finish off a front massage, but you must be careful with it if your partner is heavy .

"Never break your touch: you should always try to have at least one hand in contact with your partner's skin."

Breast massage

When you are giving your female partner a body massage, don't be afraid to include her breasts in the routine—if you omit them from it, she may be left feeling that the massage is unfinished. This simple but very sensual four-step breast massage routine was devised by the noted California masseur, Ray Stubbs.

Sideways on
A little-known fact of touch is that the sides of the breasts can feel sexier than the front areas.

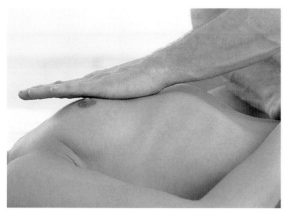

Sliding hand

Slide the flat of your right hand diagonally across her right breast, moving toward her left shoulder. Then slide your left hand across her left breast in the same manner. Repeat these two strokes alternately, about six times each.

Spiral motion

Using a well-oiled fingertip and the lightest possible touch, trace out a spiral on one of your partner's breasts. Start on the outer side and spiral in until you reach the nipple, then repeat the stroke on the other breast.

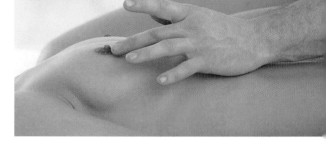

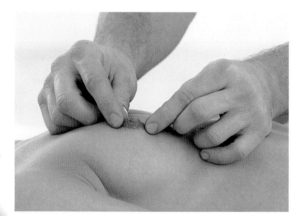

Caress nipple

Gently squeeze a little skin at each side of the nipple, and lightly slide outward as though moving along the spokes of a wheel to its rim. Repeat on all the "spokes" of each nipple.

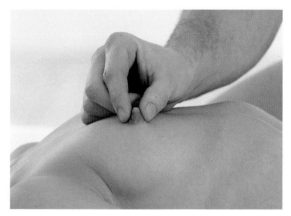

Firmer nipple slide

Squeeze the nipple gently between well-oiled forefinger and thumb, sliding them up and off it. For extra effect, use both hands alternately so that the action, and the sensations, are continuous. Repeat on the other nipple.

"The beauty of sensual touch is that when you stroke one erotic part of the body you feel the sensuality in several other sexy sites, all at the same time."

Arm massage

When I was given my first-ever massage, the practitioner included my arms and my hands as well as my back. Although I experienced less sensation in my arms than in my back, it felt utterly right that they should be included, and the hand massage was wonderful.

Arm kneading

Tuck your partner's hand into your armpit and hold the upper part of this arm with your thumbs on the top. Circle the thumbs in opposite directions, working from armpit to elbow. Lower the arm and knead down to the wrist. Repeat each stroke twice.

There are two schools of thought about the direction in which an arm massage ought to go. People who learn "lymphatic" massage, which aims to improve the circulation, work up the arm from wrist to shoulder. Those whose thoughts are directed less toward health and more toward sensuality practice kneading, stroking, and pulling down the arm, from shoulder to wrist. I have included strokes from both regimens, and I leave it up to you to decide which method suits you and your partner best. I've omitted the more vigorous of the usual arm massage strokes on the grounds that they aren't sexy enough for a sensual massage.

Massage sequence

After oiling the arms, massage one arm at a time, giving each one the complete treatment before starting on the other. Press gently if the arm is thin, more firmly if it is fleshy, but try to avoid pressing on any bones (such as at the elbow or wrist) because that can be painful. Before beginning work on your partner's other arm, you may like to make the massage feel more complete by following it with a hand massage (*see pages 96–99*).

One of the most striking parts of my own first massage was how I felt flooded with friendship and love when my experienced teacher worked on my hands. I was amazed that such simple touch was able to evoke such strong emotion. In fact, I was so knocked out by it, I became convinced that if everyone in the world had a compulsory hand massage every day of their lives, there would be no wars and no violence. This is a rather eccentric viewpoint, of course, but one that would be fascinating to try and prove. I felt such strong affection after that first massage that I could hardly bear it when the teacher at last gently withdrew his touch. I should add that this masseur started off my treatment as a complete stranger!

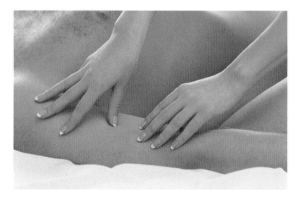

Stroking

Use your fingertips to stroke your way down your partner's arm, pressing firmly with short, overlapping strokes. Make the strokes about 4 in (10 cm) long and overlap them to create a continuous sensation. Work your way around and down the arm. Repeat twice.

OILING AND SPOILING

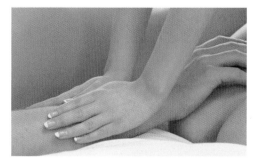

Coat the arms in oil and slide both hands up them, side by side and with palms down. Start at the wrists and end at the shoulders. Then, in a continuous movement, work down again on the insides of the arms.

Pulling

Holding the arm at the wrist, lift it straight up into the air, then pull it briefly and gently so that it stretches. Then let it relax, but without putting it down again. Repeat this light pull twice more.

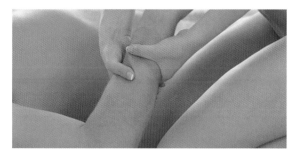

Twisting

Hold the wrists with your hands pointing in opposite directions. Then, twisting your hands in opposite directions, corkscrew your way up and down the arm, "stepping" over the elbow as you go. Your corkscrewing comes to a natural halt on the upper arm, so then work back down to the wrists. Repeat twice.

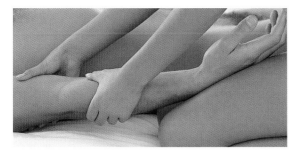

Draining

This stroke was designed to help improve circulation in the arm. Hold the arm with both hands at the wrist and thumbs on the inside of the arm. Pressing firmly with both thumbs, slowly slide them up to the elbow. Bring your thumbs back down to the wrist by drawing your hands, held flat, along the sides of the arms. Repeat.

THE ARMPIT STRETCH

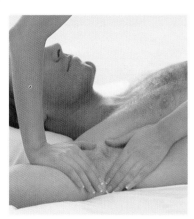

1 This is an excellent final stroke. Position your partner's arm on the ground, stretched above the head to expose the armpit. Place your hands, palms down and fingertips touching, on the armpit. With firm pressure, begin separating your hands so that the lower one slips along the side of the body and the upper glides out along the arm. Lead with the heels of your hands. Once they are clear of the armpit, move your upper hand along and gently stretch the arm. Your lower hand should curve in to the torso. Slip your hands sideways until your upper hand is at the wrist and your lower hand is near the hips.

2 Stop for a moment, holding on more tightly, and stretch your partner's arm and hip in opposite directions. Hold them stretched for a full second and then let go. Bring your hands rapidly down again to the armpit and repeat the stroke, but on ending it a second time, gently replace your partner's hand by his or her side.

Hand massage

The hands and fingers are equipped with thousands of nerve endings in every square inch of skin, which makes them very sensitive to stimuli such as touch, pressure, and temperature. Anyone who has ever cut a finger will be able to testify to the acute pain the hands can feel; what I hope to show you is the acute pleasure that can also be gained in the hands from massage.

There are many similarities between hand and foot massage, but while you are giving hand massage you are also massaging your own hand. This is, of course, true of any manual massage: your hand receives touch as it gives it. But one aspect of hand massage is like no other—it's called friendship. Hand on hand feels friendly.

Kneading

Hold your partner's hand, palm up, in both of yours. Use your thumbs to knead the fleshy parts of the palm. Cover the palm with tiny, circular strokes, pressing firmly.

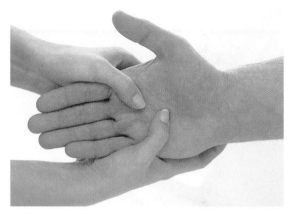

Palm and thumb massage

Use your thumb to massage the fleshy areas of your partner's palm and base of thumb. Rotate each segment of the thumb between your thumb and forefinger.

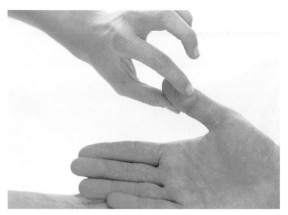

Finger manipulation

Taking your partner's thumb and each finger in turn, pull your thumb and index finger up the sides in short, twisting strokes. On reaching the tip, work down again.

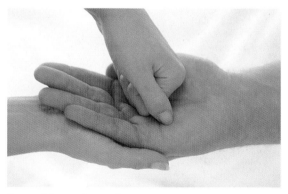

Knuckling the palm

Press your knuckles into the palm of your partner's hand just below the fingers. Then scrape your knuckles from side to side, working your way toward the wrist.

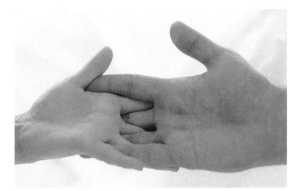

Finger lacing

Lace your fingers through your partner's, palms up. Press against the back of your partner's hand so that the palm is flexed upward. Flex, then relax, three times.

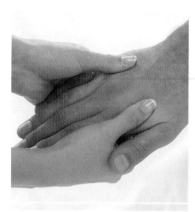

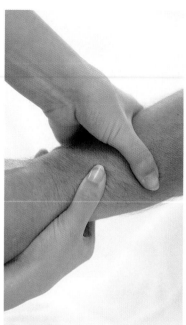

Circling the wrist

Encircle your partner's wrist with thumb and forefinger, then lightly twist these several times from side to side around the wrist.

Circling the backs

Holding your partner's hand at each side, use both thumbs to circle all over the back of the hand, including the wrist. Massage with a firm but gentle pressure.

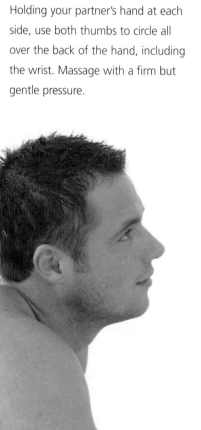

In the groove

Firmly holding onto your partner's hand with one of your hands, run the thumbpad of your other hand down each of the grooves between the tendons on the back of his or her hand. Start at the wrist and finish at the fingers.

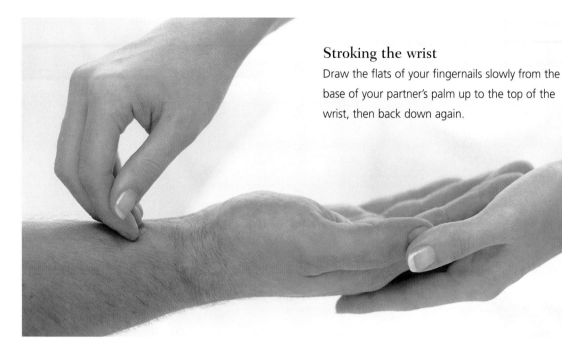

Stroking the wrist

Draw the flats of your fingernails slowly from the base of your partner's palm up to the top of the wrist, then back down again.

"One aspect of hand massage is like no other—it's called friendship. Hand on hand feels friendly."

Finishing off

Hold your partner's hand between both of yours. Breathe deeply and imagine that your hands are sending energy into your partner.

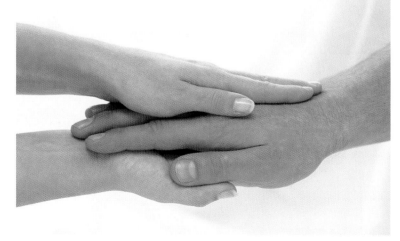

Leg massage

Completing a task is as important as beginning it, and how you complete something often reflects your personality. If you're an impatient character, you might skimp the ending, to get the job over and done with quickly. But if you're a thoughtful personality, you might make the ending as lingering and as tactile as you did the start, and this is the approach to adopt for the leg massage, the final stage of a full-body massage. Here are the massage strokes for the backs of the legs; those for the fronts are on pages 103–05.

Oiling and spoiling
Starting at the ankle, work up to the buttocks and then down again. Place your hands one above the other, with fingers in opposite directions, and slide them up the thigh.

If you skip massaging your partner's legs during your whole-body session, it will make the entire session less than satisfactory. And your partner might wonder why you chose to ignore them. And instead of ending up feeling relaxed, sensual, even ecstatic, your partner might instead feel let down, which would be a pity after all the hard work on your part.

When you massage the backs of your partner's legs, he or she should lie face down. Using a similar stroke to the one with which you oiled the arms (*see page 93*), begin by massaging oil into the backs of the legs, one leg at a time.

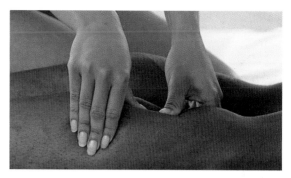

Draining

Place your hands around the ankle, with the thumbs pointing in opposite directions. Slide your hands up to the knee, pressing firmly with your thumbs and fingers. Then work down, with the same position but with no pressure.

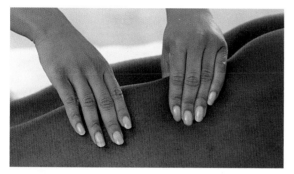

Kneading

Use the kneading stroke here that was used for the hips (*see page 79*). Work down from the thighs, kneading only the fleshy areas; omit the backs of the knees.

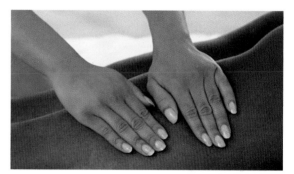

Deep-pressure circling

Pressing the palms of your hands on the back of the leg, rotate the skin and the flesh below it in small circles. Do this on the fleshy areas only, and do not press too hard.

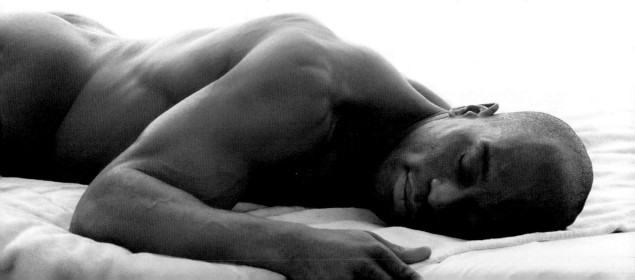

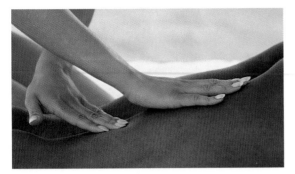

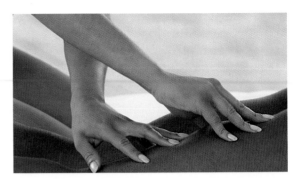

Hand over hand

Starting at the thigh, draw one hand down 4 in (10 cm), then repeat with the other hand. Cover the whole of the back of each leg, working downward only.

Deep finger pressure

This is basically the same as the hand-over-hand stroke but, instead of using all of your hand, simply press firmly with your fingertips. Again, work downward only.

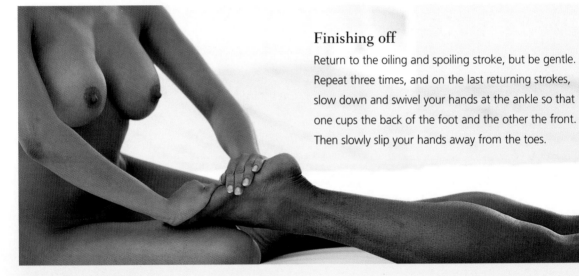

Finishing off

Return to the oiling and spoiling stroke, but be gentle. Repeat three times, and on the last returning strokes, slow down and swivel your hands at the ankle so that one cups the back of the foot and the other the front. Then slowly slip your hands away from the toes.

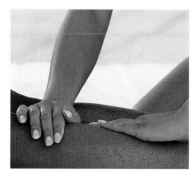

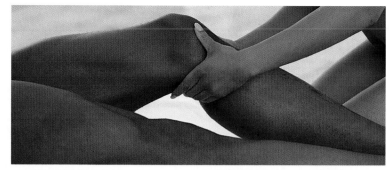

Oiling and spoiling

Using a similar stroke to oiling the arms *(see page 93)*, work the oil into the fronts of the legs. Sweep your hands, palms down, fingers pointing in opposite directions and one hand placed above the other, up the front of each leg. Reduce the pressure when you pass over the kneecap, and continue up to the abdomen.

Kneecapping

This is much gentler than it sounds. Intertwine your fingers at the back of the knee, and then lightly circle the edge of the kneecap with the tips of your thumbs.

Return strokes

When you bring your hands down again during oiling, separate them to each side of the leg and sweep them smoothly down in one long, sensuous, uninterrupted move.

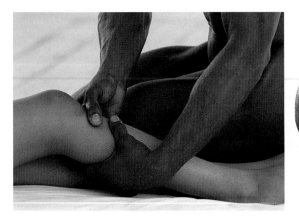

Under friction

Instead of circling the kneecap with your thumbs, place them both just below it, press them in, and slide them rhythmically together and apart like opposing pistons.

Kneading

Concentrating on the thigh only, knead the area with both hands, as you did when kneading the hips *(see page 79)* and the backs of the legs. Give each handful of flesh a gentle twisting motion as you squeeze. When you get used to the kneading action, you will be able to squeeze the flesh so that it appears to travel from one hand to the other with a short, wavelike motion.

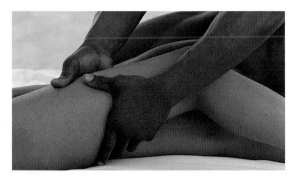

Draining

The fronts of the thighs are where the draining stroke is at its most effective. Use the same stroke as for the backs of the thighs *(see page 101)* and don't be afraid to use firm pressure. Avoid this stroke below the knees because it can feel uncomfortable, and don't put any pressure on the kneecaps.

Hand over hand

Use the same technique as for the backs of the legs *(see page 102)*. With a light touch, begin by being quick and brisk and then make it slow and sensuous.

"Never forget to massage extra slowly so that your strokes are experienced as timeless."

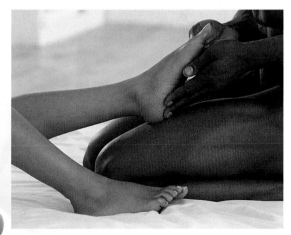

Finishing off

When massaging your partner's legs, end with a hand-over-hand stroke at the foot. You might then try a foot massage *(see page 35).*

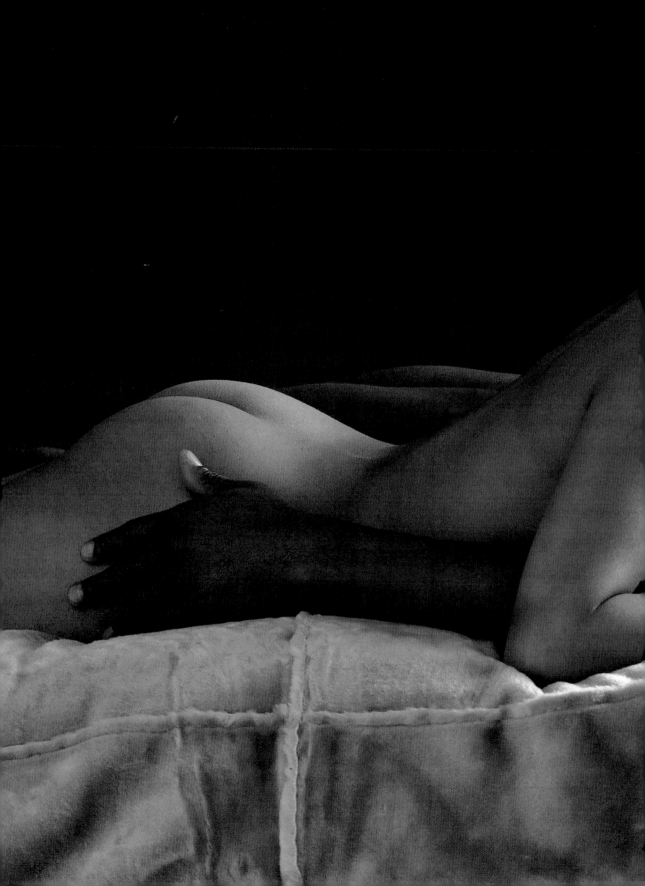

Intimate massage

4

Eroticism

What makes an erotic moment? Is it an unexpected move or proposition? Is it the forbidden? Can any touch be found erotic? Or does it have to be made with a specific intent? Perhaps each person has his or her own definition of what is erotic, and that definition is unique to that individual.

Sensual massage
This is a wonderful form of foreplay, and can provide the high levels of arousal that some women need to help them reach orgasm.

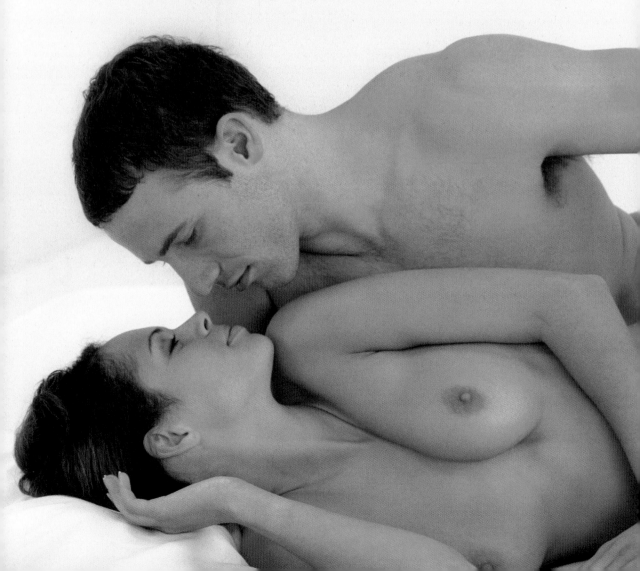

But there's a difference between eroticism, lust, and even passion. If boy meets girl, and they experience instant attraction, even if they hurl themselves into the bedroom and feel quite savage with desire, it is not necessarily an erotic situation. The very breath of eroticism contains leisureliness. It involves thought, deliberation, and losing yourself in a sensual landscape. It's where an unexpected proposition or move might well be erotic because it puts sensual ideas into your head. And yes, the forbidden may be part of eroticism, but it's not the whole. For when you have glimpsed the sexual idea that is erotic, the manner in which this idea is then translated into real lovemaking often falls short of the thought.

Masturbation and eroticism

Think of the man or woman who masturbates to pornography. He or she may enjoy a rich fantasy life and have wonderfully powerful orgasms. But this is not erotic because there is no element of the unknown, no other person to inject a special quality into the lovemaking, no uncertainty, and therefore no certainty either.

Without these things we miss out on having trust in the other, confidence about oneself, and a liberating sense of openness in which we feel we can do anything and it will all be wonderful.

Erotic relationships

That's all very well, you might say, but how do you bring eroticism into an already established relationship, where you've been making love for years? It's not surprising if you feel erotic with someone new, but what if you have the aging-relationship factor to contend with?

Perhaps the key is being open to new ideas, because new ideas help us to develop mentally. This means you and your partner being truly honest about the state of your relationship, even if such honesty is risky. It may mean accepting that lovemaking has become dull, and that you need to try something different.

For her pleasure

First moves
Before you begin the massage of your partner's genitals, lovingly stroke and pleasure the rest of her body. Approach her genitals along the inside of her thigh, itself a highly sensitive area.

This massage, and the following one for men (*see pages 114–17*), is based on methods taught by Ray Stubbs, and by graduates of the Institute for the Advanced Study of Human Sexuality in San Francisco. It should only be included after the rest of your partner's body has been pleasured.

While all of the strokes for men came complete with title, none of the strokes for women were named, so I have given them names myself.

The idea of the gentle hair torture is not, of course, torture, but to cause exquisite pricking sensations that travel from the mons pubis straight to that delicate sex organ, the clitoris. It consists of systematically tugging small individual tufts of pubic hair.

The duck's bill is experienced by the woman as a flooding sensation, full of warmth but slightly disturbing—which is as it should be. Holding your hand pointing downward, in a kind of duck's bill shape, pour warm massage oil slowly over the hand so that it falls in a thin stream onto her clitoris.

Wibbling has its origins in childlike play. As children, many of us pull the bottom lip of the mouth down and then let go. If you do this quickly and often, it makes a "wibble" sound. Try it for yourself, then when you have gotten the hang of it you can do some "genital wibbling" on your partner. Start with one of the outer labia (lips) of her vagina, gently pulling it and letting it go in a rhythmic manner. Begin at the lower end and work your way up to the clitoris. When you've wibbled one outer lip, repeat the process on the other, and then move on to the inner lips.

For clitoral maneuvers, use a lubricated finger to circle the head of the clitoris lightly at a steady pace. Then change direction and circle in the opposite direction. After 20 or so circles each way, rub the tip of your finger lightly up and down the side of the clitoris, 20 times on each side. Now rub backward and forward immediately below the clitoris 20 times. Finally, rub from the clitoris down to the opening of the vagina and back 20 times.

There are many variations on all these strokes, and you might like to invent your own. But always ensure that your partner and your fingers are adequately oiled.

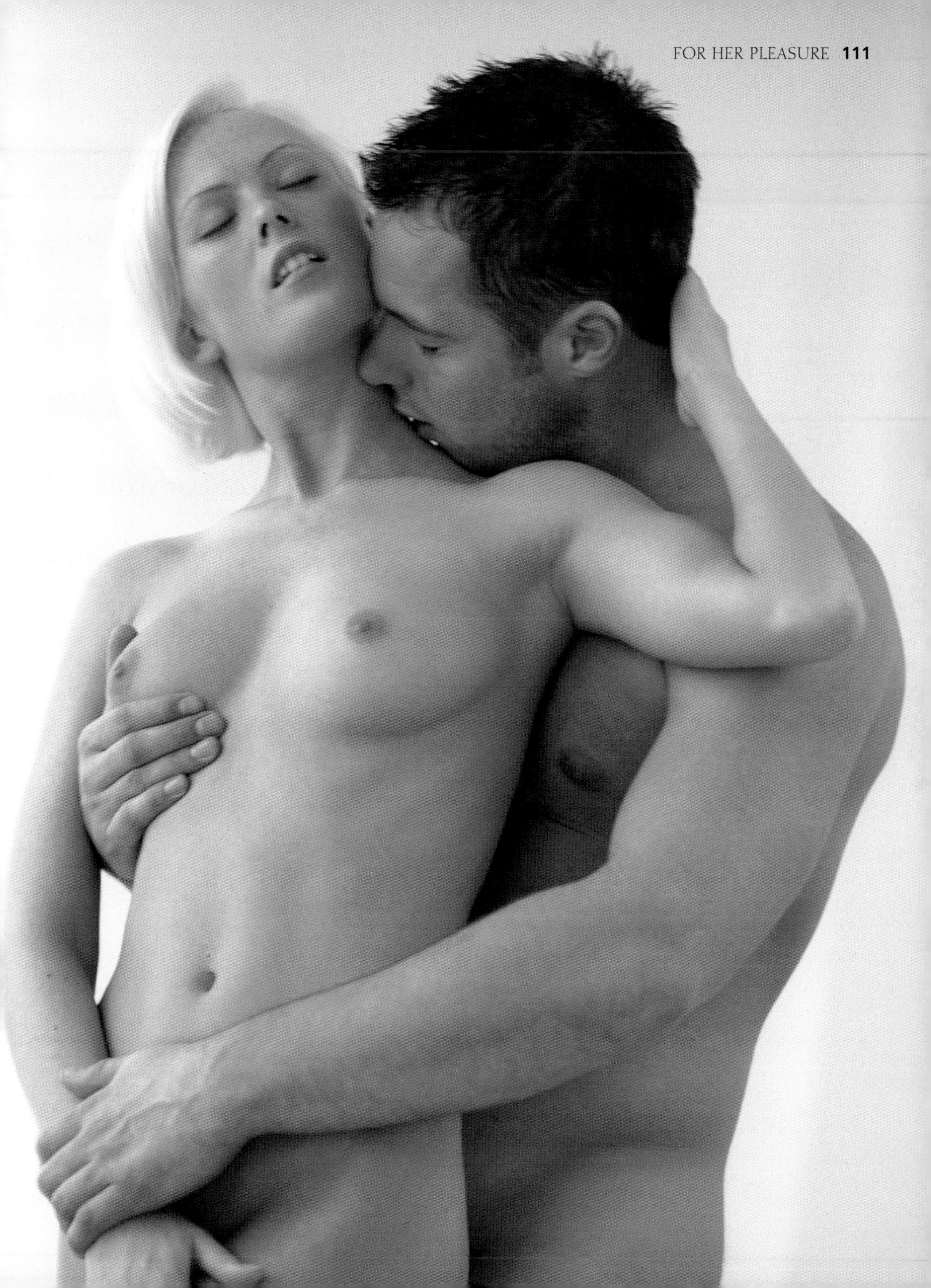

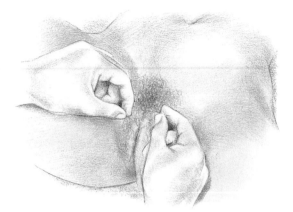

The gentle hair torture

Pull her pubic hair, gently and in small
tufts. Using both hands at a time,
work your way slowly from the
top of her pubic hair and
down each side of the labia.

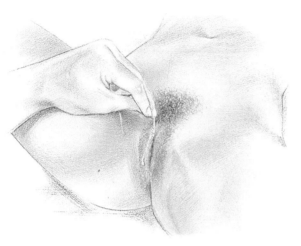

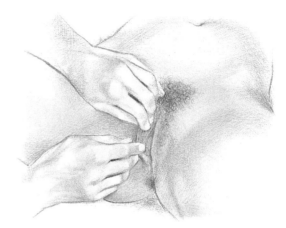

Duck's bill

Shape the fingers of one hand into a "duck's bill," hold them above her clitoris, and pour warmed massage oil over them so that it slowly seeps through and runs onto her genitals.

Wibbling

Start with one of the outer labia. Use both your hands at the same time, gently pull on it, then let go, just as you might do if this were one of the lips of your mouth.

Highly aroused

Intimate massage can be used as a sensational finale to a sensual massage, as a highly arousing form of foreplay, or simply for the pleasure that it provides.

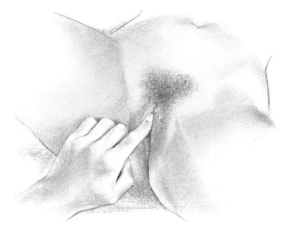

Clitoral maneuvers

Extremely delicately, with an almost featherlight touch and using plenty of lubrication, run your finger first around the head and then up and down the shaft of her clitoris.

For his pleasure

When giving your man genital massage, remember that you are not aiming at bringing him to orgasm. If it happens, it's a bonus for him, but if not, it really doesn't matter, because you will still have given him wonderful sensations. These are the basic strokes I was originally taught, but there is nothing to prevent you from inventing a few of your own.

The build-up

A genital massage only works fully when it is preceded by an all-over body massage. It is important *not* to stint on this preliminary.

As with the massage for her pleasure (*see pages 110–13*), this ideally should not be used without massaging the rest of the body first; it isn't nearly as effective without that whole-body build-up. Begin by pouring a little warm oil into your hands and then liberally applying this to your partner's genitals, ensuring that his penis, testicles, and perineum are covered. Since this is a hairy area, use enough oil to allow your hands to slide around without catching.

The countdown

This consists of two strokes. For the first, grasp the top of his penis with your right hand and place your left hand underneath his testicles, with fingers positioned toward the anus. As you slide your right hand down the penile shaft, enclosing it as much as possible, bring your left hand up from his testicles. Aim to bring both hands slowly together at the base of the shaft.

For the second stroke, slide your right hand back up his penis from the base while simultaneously bringing your left hand back under his testicles again. Again, work slowly and steadily.

This is the basis of the countdown, with which you then go on to overwhelm your partner. The count goes as follows:

- 10 times the first stroke, then 10 times the second
- nine times the first stroke, then nine times the second
- eight times the first stroke then eight times the second, and so on until you reach one stroke.

Be inviting
Use the whole of your body to arouse your man and get him into a receptive mood.

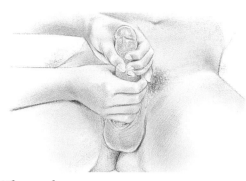

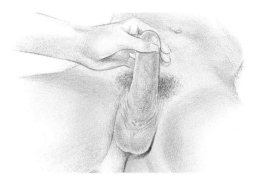

The corkscrew

This basically involves rubbing the shaft of his penis between your palms. Do this gently, but maintain fairly firm pressure. Put one hand on each side of the penis shaft. Slide them around in opposite directions at the same time—as if you were trying to twist the penis in half—and then slide them back again. Repeat 10 times.

The squeeze technique

This is used to control ejaculation. If your partner tells you that he has the urge to ejaculate, grasp his penis and press your thumb against it just below the glans. Maintain firm pressure for 10 seconds, or until his urge to ejaculate has subsided. If he then loses his erection, use your massage methods to get it back.

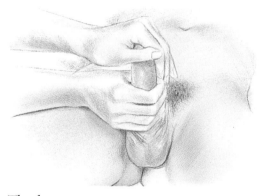

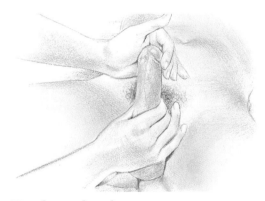

The lemon squeezer

In this stroke, steady the penis by grasping it around the halfway mark with one hand. Then rub the cupped palm of your other hand over and around the head of the penis, as if you were juicing a lemon. It helps if you close your eyes and actually feel your hand brushing across the surface. Circle very gently, moving your hand first 10 times clockwise and then a further 10 times counterclockwise. Use steady strokes, rather than slow ones, and as you become adept at making them, you will find that they take on a particular rhythm.

Hand over hand

Like the simple children's game of "hand over hand," where you repeatedly bring your hand from underneath the pile of hands and place it on top, never breaking the rhythm, this has to be performed pretty quickly. Slide your cupped hand over the head and down the shaft. Before it gets to the base, bring the other hand up to the head to repeat the stroke. The goal is to keep up a continuous hand-over-hand movement so that the head of his penis remains uncovered for as little time as possible.

Sex in the brain

The brain is perhaps the most powerful sex organ of all, because sexual thoughts can create physical sensations. Men are able to achieve an erection and some women climax simply by fantasizing about an attractive person.

Men and women whose sexual feelings have been dormant for years may find that their sexual responses blossom as the result of a chance encounter with someone whose imagination triggers theirs. Suddenly they're feeling like teenagers again because, for the first time in years, someone matches, indeed challenges, the far shores of their own fantasy worlds.

Our fantasy lives often begin with dreams, frequently the first occasions on which boys and some girls reach climax. Afterward, we may remember the dream and unconsciously re-create the sexual scene within it. It is our first experience of fantasizing. As our sexual sophistication increases, so too does the content of our fantasies. If we're lucky, we may find ourselves able to recount these fantasies to our lovers. Perhaps they, too, may be turned on by them, and help embellish the ideas so that we end up creating sexual stories jointly with our lovers.

Erotic scenarios

Using fantasy to transport yourself into an erotic scenario is an easy way to improve the quality of a sexual experience.

FANTASY AS COMPENSATION

Fantasy may be used unconsciously to compensate for imbalance in our daily lives. For instance, a judge may need the occasional break from his power and responsibility by being treated like a slave or an infant. His sexual fantasies may provide such an escape. A woman who has had powerful restrictions placed upon her expression of her sexuality may need to imagine being overpowered before she can respond fully to arousal. There is also an opposite case, where a woman who is powerful at work needs her partner to expose her inner frailties. But if he is unable to, she might then take refuge in dreams of seduction.

Sexual fantasies can be very beneficial to both men and women, whether they are used as a prelude to lovemaking, during intercourse, or during mutual or solo masturbation. They can, for instance, be used to revitalize a sexual relationship that has grown stale and boring. They can also sometimes be of help to men with erectile problems, and to women who have difficulty becoming fully aroused.

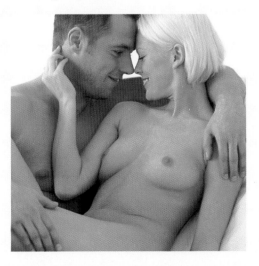

The use of fantasy

When I worked for *Penthouse Forum*, many of the sexual exploits described in readers' letters were obviously fake, but some of them were borderline. We would invariably include these letters because, even if the experiences were fantasies, such fantasies were, we figured, legitimate aspects of sexuality.

Restraint fantasies
A common theme in sexual fantasies is that of being physically restrained in some way.

But what about people who don't have sexual fantasies? I meet some of them in my women's sexuality workshops. These workshops are for women who so far are unable to experience orgasm. Many are helped by learning to fantasize, which they do by reading sexy literature and then, next time they are making love, visualizing the stories that aroused them. Other women in the same groups need only to be "given permission" to fantasize, and turn out to be able to do so without the help of books.

Using fantasies

Many people prefer to keep their fantasies for their own private use, because then they remain entirely personal. In addition, some people are very ashamed of their fantasies, while others fear that a fantasy will lose its eroticism if aired in public. A lot of people, however, like to talk their fantasies through with a partner. Doing this can be such an act of trust that the relationship deepens.

Another advantage shows up when you discover that your partner has corresponding or complementary fantasies. In these circumstances, your fantasies may be enriched and grow in eroticism, and can be used to develop sensational sex and remarkable love.

GOING FURTHER

Going even further and actually acting out a fantasy can be a powerfully exciting adjunct to your sex life. There are many men and women who have played out fantasies such as picking each other up in bars, visiting hotel rooms wearing only fur coats, and making love outdoors. It's something to do with taking a risk in public. If you know that underneath your coat you are naked, it's very arousing to cross the hotel lobby. As long as these activities don't infringe on anyone else's privacy, don't harm anyone, and don't break any laws, they can be amazingly stimulating.

The option to refuse

It is, of course, important to remember that if you feel you are being asked to do something that feels wrong, you should not hesitate to refuse. Also, it is a reasonable general rule that if your fantasy, or your partner's fantasy, involves any kind of violence, leave it well alone.

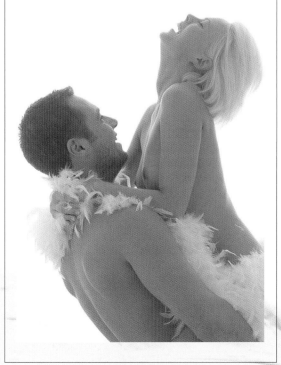

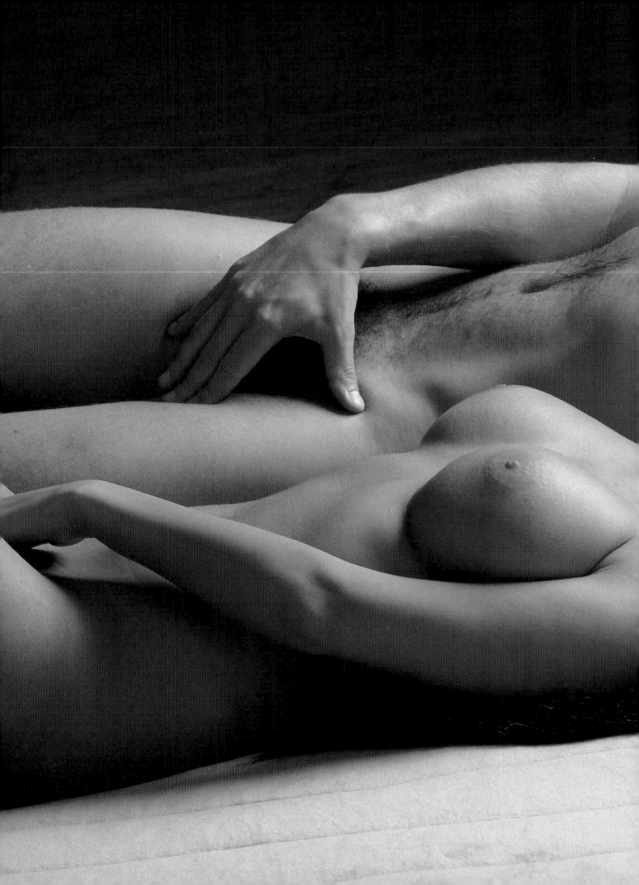

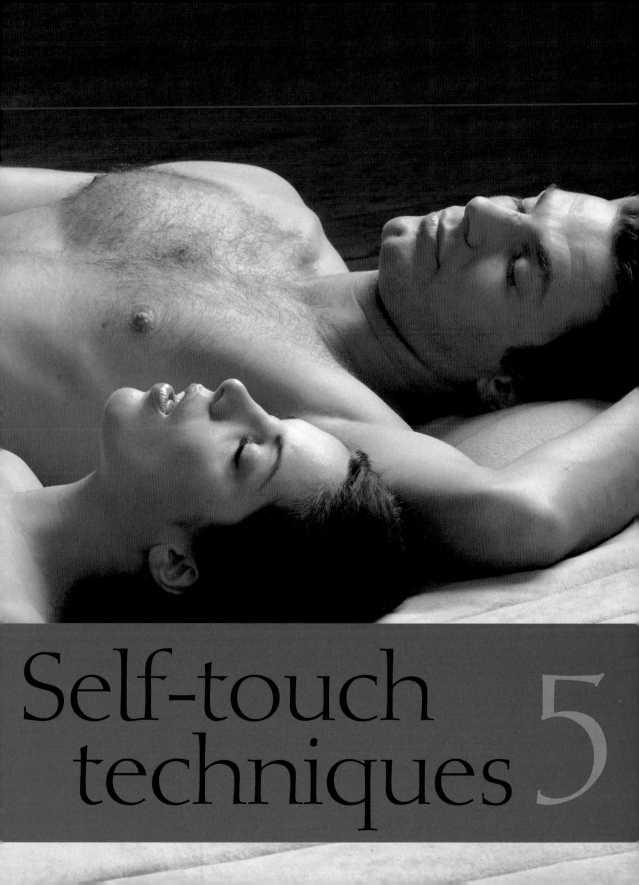

Self-touch techniques 5

Using self-touch

Not everyone has a partner, and some of us prefer to live alone. This does not mean that we want to be starved of sensual touch, nor that we lose our sensuality or the desire to develop as sexual beings. In these situations a sensual self-touch routine can help us maintain our sexuality, but it can also be used to enhance a relationship.

As we grow up, we consciously identify our sexual needs as well as unconsciously crave closeness, and we learn to look for specific sexual sensations—men more so than women. Because their genitals are so easy to find, and because they so naturally learn how to stimulate themselves, men usually develop their genital sensation as the main focus of their sensuality.

This means that when it comes to building a physical relationship with a woman, male genital sensation often comes into conflict with female all-over body sensation. It's important to say here that neither is "right": men and women have different routes to sexual development.

One of the great benefits of this difference in sexual focus is that, as we become more educated about sex, we can learn from each other. We can deliberately set out to gain new sexual perspectives from our partners that enrich our own sensual lives and increase our mutual enjoyment of lovemaking.

Self-touch for women

In the sexuality workshops I used to hold for women, most of the participants—ranging in age from 17 to 60—attended because they had never experienced an orgasm. A number of common denominators were observed: ignorance of the body, the genitals, and sexual response; a shared sense of isolation; and a lack of confidence. By working even on only one of these issues, their lives improved immeasurably.

The methods I used were based on a mixture of group therapy styles developed in the US by Lonnie Barbach and also by Betty Dodson. Betty was my main influence, and the self-touch techniques for women that I describe are my own interpretation of Betty's inspired routines.

Self-touch for men

Men in the Western world are often starved of touch from an early age. There is the misbelief that this is part of a "toughening-up" process to prepare boys for the cruel outside world, but this way of thinking is flawed. In many Eastern cultures, men have traditionally been allowed far more sensuality as boys than they have in the West. Yet they survived and were still masculine enough to beget children. Lack of touch is definitely not necessary to modern life.

On the following pages, therefore, I propose a self-loving routine to help men use the whole body as an erogenous zone and thus further whole-body responses. This should extend your sensuality and enrich your life.

Exploring sexuality

We can enlarge our sexual horizons on our own. We can explore new aspects of sensuality for our own pleasure, and by developing sides to sexual selves that are more commonly ascribed to the opposite sex, we are likely to become better lovers.

Self-touch for men

For this routine, arrange to have at least an hour of uninterrupted privacy. Begin by giving yourself a warm bath or shower. A bath is preferable since it is a more relaxing experience and brings us closer to the days when we were floating in our mothers' wombs.

Preparation
Ensure that you have absolute privacy, and begin by taking a warm bath to relax. This relaxation will help to clear your mind of outside troubles so that you can concentrate on, and enjoy, the self-touch routine that follows.

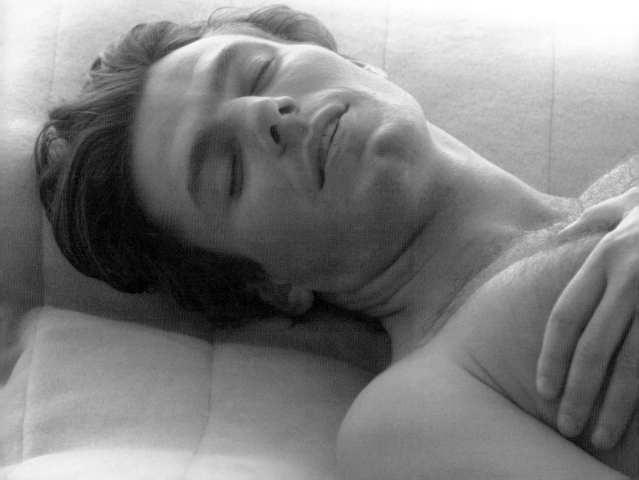

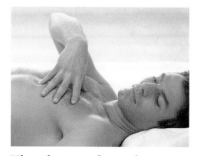

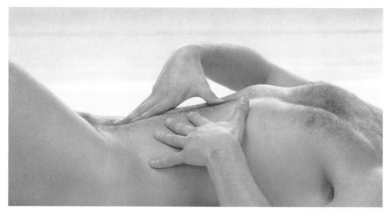

The chest and nipples

Apply the massage oil with both hands and move them in circles all over your chest except on the nipples, covering a small area at a time. Then apply a little fresh oil to each of your nipples and gently stroke, squeeze, and fondle them to find out what it feels like. Close your eyes and imagine that it's a beautiful woman who's stimulating you.

The abdomen

This is an area where many people are ticklish, but even the most ticklish can be tamed by the use of a firm touch. Oil your hands and move them firmly in circles over your abdomen, repeatedly working down from your waist to your groin and back up again. Once you've relaxed beneath your firm touch you may then surprise yourself by being able to enjoy a lighter one, so repeat the stroke, using a lighter action. Using forefingers, try pressing down deep in order to massage the colon, counterclockwise.

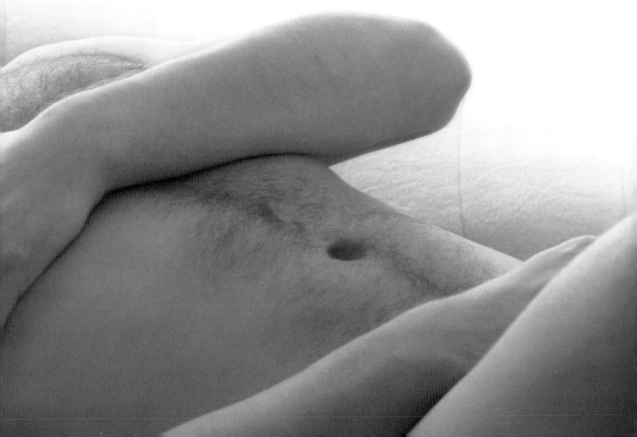

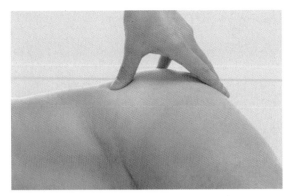

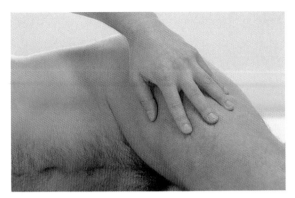

The buttocks

Lie on your side or your belly and rub oil onto your buttocks with your fingertips, using large, circular, swirling movements. Note any sensation near the anus and the perineum. If it were your lover caressing you, how would you like her to do it? Imagine you are her and direct your hands accordingly. Don't be afraid to let your fingers linger on the sexy spots!

The thighs

Stroke repeatedly the area from your knees up to your genitals, covering both the outsides and the insides of your thighs. When you massage your thighs, note the level of touch that feels most arousing, and as you continue touching, build on the erotic pricklings and see if you can enlarge these sensations without yet touching your genitals.

The hands and arms

Begin by pouring a little warmed oil into your hands and massaging it from one hand to the other. Next, massage the back of each hand, noting the texture you are touching, then move on to your arms. Use powerful strokes up and down each arm, then squeeze the arm by the wrist, and push your hand up to the elbow. Follow these firm strokes with more gentle touching.

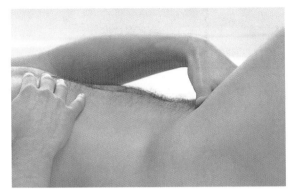

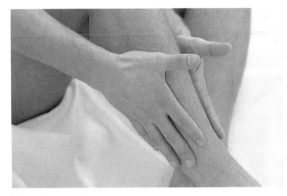

The penis

Lie on your back, propped against the pillows. As you stroke your penis, imagine your lover. Would she manipulate your foreskin? Or rub your scrotum? Would she hold your penis harder than you do? Try speeding up your stroke without making it harder, then slowing down but grasping more firmly. As you end in orgasm, continue to visualize your woman's hands around you.

The lower leg

Stroke each leg, in turn, working from the ankle up to the knee and back. The foot is one of the most fertile areas for self-massage. When you are working on your feet, you will find that it is possible to use most of the basic foot-massage techniques that you would normally use on your partner *(see pages 36–37)*. Pay special attention to those erogenous zones between the toes.

"You are attempting, by caressing your body, to bring to life nerve endings that have hardly been used."

Self-touch for women

This erotic self-touch routine is a highly pleasurable way of exploring your own body and getting to know and love it. By indulging yourself in such an intimate and sensuous fashion, you will be discovering your own likes and dislikes when it comes to sensual touch.

Loving your body

Admire your naked body. If you are a plump woman, be proud of your curves; if you are thin and wiry, appreciate your delicate figure and the strength that it possesses.

Begin by treasuring yourself. This sounds embarrassingly corny and therefore difficult to do, but it's worth trying. Look at yourself in a mirror and say, out loud, "I love you." Then embellish this: tell yourself, "You're terrific and I think you're wonderful." And look at yourself as if you love yourself, perhaps by smiling, or by looking seductive or passionate. And when, in the future, you start being hard on yourself, stop for a minute, give yourself a hug, and say, "You're OK. I love you." Try to do this exercise two or three times a day for a month—you'll be pleasantly surprised at how much better you begin to feel.

A sensual shower

Give yourself a treat in the comforting warmth of a good shower. Lather yourself sensuously with your favorite shower gel and imagine it is your lover's hands that are doing the touching. He thinks your body is wonderful and his hands roam lovingly over your soapy crevices.

Now that he has cornered you and is touching your genitals, let yourself go with whatever moves your hands choose to make as they slide across your genitals, making them more and more slippery and sensitive. Sometimes they go slowly and sometimes their movements get very fast indeed. Have fun being your own lover.

Self-massage

Go in for this as if it were a massage with a partner. Prepare the room so that it provides you with a sensual background (*see page 75*). If you can, position yourself in front of a mirror so that you see your oily hands lightly sliding across your body and exploring your own contours.

Be aware of areas of tense muscle and try to wriggle and relax them. Massage them firmly if it helps, letting your body yield to the pressure of your hands. If tension persists, try relieving it with the tense/relax method, which involves tensing your muscles hard for a count of five before letting go again. Relax the muscles in your face and mouth, and wriggle your neck, your arms, and your waist to make sure that all of these are loosened up.

Then begin your massage, starting at your head. Slowly rub, circle, and knead your way down to your chest and breasts, then work your way down your abdomen and pass on to your thighs, legs, and feet.

In your foot massage, use your thumbs and knuckles when you are working on the soles, and the tips of your thumbs when massaging between the tendons on the tops of the feet. Remember to include your toes in your foot massage.

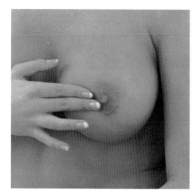

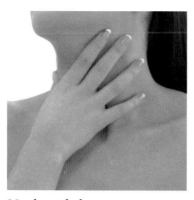

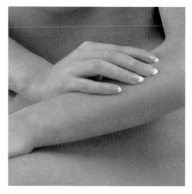

Nipples

Coat your nipples and areolae with massage oil and, using your fingertips, trace delicate circles on and around them.

Neck and throat

Give your hands a generous coating of oil, then gently stroke, fondle, and caress your neck and throat with your fingers and fingertips, and with the palms of your hands.

Arms

Pour a little oil into your hands and coat your forearms with it. Work it well into the skin, using powerful strokes, then stroke your forearms gently and lovingly with your fingers. Repeat on your upper arms.

Breasts

With warm, well-oiled hands, fondle and caress your breasts and move them in circles, paying attention to the bottoms and sides as well as to the tops and fronts. Then gently knead and squeeze them, first one at a time and then both together. Note which kind of touch feels best.

Buttocks

While lying on your front or side, stroke your buttocks with your fingertips and the palms of your hands, then gently knead them.

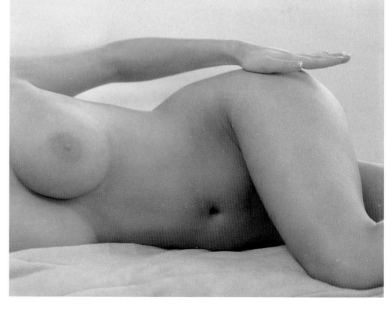

Insides of the thighs

After massaging your buttocks, roll over onto your back and, without touching your genitals, stroke and fondle the insides of your thighs.

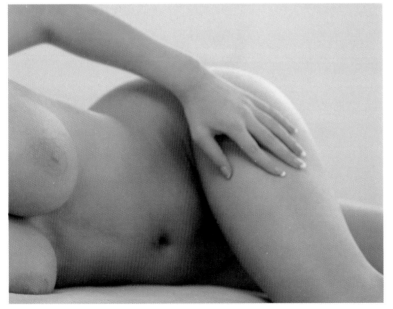

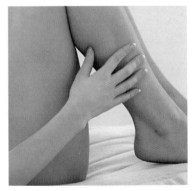

Calves

Lie on your back and run your hands up the backs and sides of your calves, squeezing them gently with your fingers and thumbs.

Outsides of the thighs

Roll onto one side and massage the outside of your uppermost thigh. Then roll onto your other side and repeat on the other thigh.

Genital pleasuring

Move last to your genitals, massaging them in the same way that you did the rest of your body. Try looking at them in a mirror. Can you visualize them as a flower? Is it possible to arrange your labia into a flower shape?

Now spread your labia back so that you can see inside. Can you identify your clitoris and the hood around it, and below it the tiny urethra and the entrance to your vagina? Gently place your finger inside your vagina and note the texture of its interior. Can you reach to the far end where you can touch the tip of your cervix? Can you find the G-spot, which is thought to be located on the front wall of the vagina, some way toward the far end?

Try moving your finger around the inside of your vagina. Note where there is more feeling and where there is less. Put your finger at the 12 o'clock position (near the clitoris) and crook it slightly. How does this feel? Try running your fingertip around the entrance to the vagina.

Now move your lubricated finger up to your clitoris and see if you prefer the finger circling on the clitoral head itself, or around it, or on either side. Or perhaps you like it on all these spots?

Continue with your genital exploration and build on the good sensations—the goal is to make connections between your brain and your genitals that are strictly pleasurable. You might like to enhance your stimulation by using a vibrator, but if, with fingers or vibrator, you feel yourself approaching climax, stave it off—try to keep on the brink for about 15 to 30 minutes.

Genitals

Finally, lovingly caress and fondle your genitals. Explore them with your fingers, starting with the labia and vagina and then moving on to stimulate your clitoris.

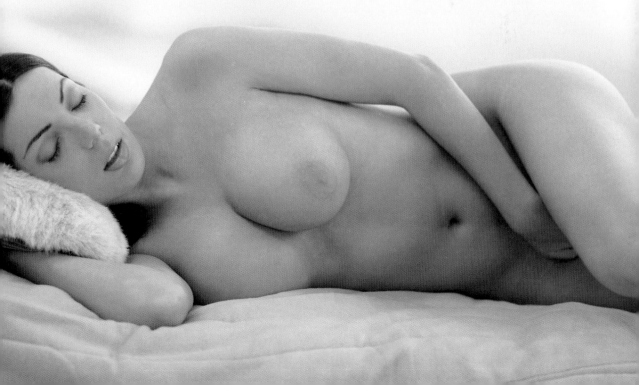

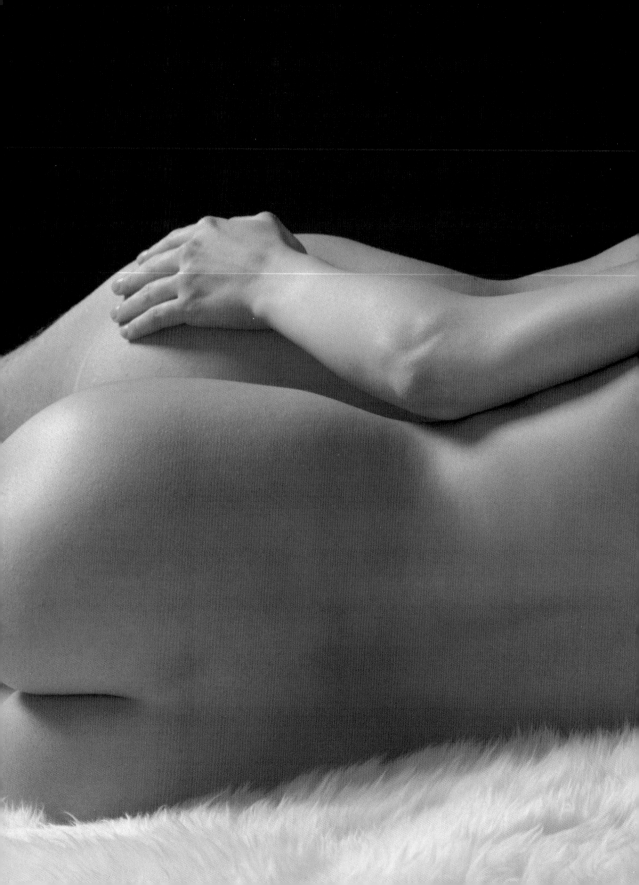

Touch for life changes 6

Touch for life changes

For many years, sex researchers have been trying to discover the exact nature of sexual desire, and to find out why, so often, it does not last. These questions have yet to be answered, but we do know that flagging interest in sex can often be overcome by using sensual touch.

A stronger relationship

When you work together to overcome the difficulties created by life changes, you can strengthen the bonds of love that underpin your relationship.

The difficulty with living in a fast-moving, urbanized technological society is that we tend to lose touch with the natural rhythms of life. For example, because we have central heating and air conditioning to keep us comfortable, and freezers in which to store our food all year round, we are much less affected by the changes of the seasons than our ancestors were. Unfortunately, being able to distance ourselves from the external rhythms of nature has also led us to try ignoring our internal rhythms and patterns, particularly those that are related to growing older.

As little children, we are blessed with a store of apparently boundless energy. That energy takes on different but hectic patterns in adolescence, remains abundant in our 20s, and starts to wind down when we reach our late 30s. By the time we reach 50, we may still feel young inside, but parts of our body just don't work in the ways they used to. And when we reach old age, unless we have—exceptionally—kept fit, we are most likely to be slow and stiff.

I'm stating the obvious here for one very good reason, and that is that no one ever expects the aging process to be reflected in his or her sex life (although many people think, erroneously, that sexual activity ceases in old age). Few people make allowances for the fact that ill-health and old age affect our sexual capabilities, as do (for women) pregnancy, nursing a baby, menstruation, and menopause.

Lack of desire

There are times in our lives when it is perfectly normal not to feel sexual desire, not to want to take part in the sex act, and not to need any sexual release. There is nothing wrong in feeling these things when there are good reasons to do so. They do not mean that we are lacking or wanting in any way, and it's a tragedy that we have somehow come to think we are.

Sensual response

The response that doesn't change and remains steadfast throughout these sexual fluctuations is the sensual one. If you are someone who, on feeling the touch of a lover's hand, reacts with sensuality, you will probably continue to do so regardless of your age and the state of your health. Indeed, because touch is comforting as well as sensual, we probably need it far more than we need sex.

TOUCH PATTERNS

Touch patterns and rites can help us through some of the more tricky stages of life. These will not, however, work effectively if they are used in isolation. If they are to be of any real value, you should combine them with the kind of basic, everyday loving touch that helps to keep any relationship on track.

In addition, if your partner is going through a major life change, he or she is liable to feelings of uncertainty and insecurity. You may need to show a great deal of sympathy and understanding, which you should always combine with good, old-fashioned, tender loving care.

Menstruation

Between the ages of about 13 and 50, women are subject to monthly menstrual cycles, undergoing the physical manifestations of ovulation and of shedding the lining of the uterus. This is accompanied by changes in hormone levels, and since women's moods are affected by hormones, it means that women tend to experience emotions on a cyclical basis, too.

The best way to discover just what your monthly emotional pattern consists of is to keep a menstruation diary. Over two or three months, chart not just the physical changes you notice during menstruation but the emotional ones too, noting on which day in the cycle they occur. This will show you how your moods alter during your menstrual cycle. When you can predict how you will be feeling you can, if necessary, alter your behavior to compensate for it.

Menstruation and touch

The hormonal fluctuations of menstruation can affect how a woman experiences touch, and my diary highlighted this. It showed that for 24 hours before my menses, my skin felt fantastic, and every tiny touch thrilled through me—this touch was better than the climax when it arrived. During the first 12 or so days of each menstrual month, I was relaxed, full of energy, and highly sexual. Then, for 48 hours, I would be extremely tired, probably due to my body ovulating at the time.

Afterward, I got more irritable as the end of the menstrual month approached, and though I could feel sexual and have orgasms, I wouldn't initiate sex. Yet when I was at my touchiest, around Day 26, I would revert to being highly sexual. Though it was a shock to realize that for almost the full second half of my menstrual month I was not particularly interested in sex, seeing this pattern enabled me to become calmer and more sure of myself.

Menstrual symptoms

Hormonal changes in the second half of the menstrual cycle can cause a number of adverse effects, such as headaches and tender breasts. For relaxing warmth, ask your partner to cuddle you in a "spoons" position.

"Recent European studies show women commonly feel at their most sensual immediately before menstruation."

BUILDING ON SENSITIVITY

Relaxation

Paradoxically, by increasing tension you can eventually relax. A long swim or a jog that uses up all your spare energy will help. If you don't enjoy physical exercise, a good alternative is to put yourself through the tense/relax exercise *(see page 25)*.

Physical warmth

Many women (but not all) find that experiencing physical warmth helps them to relax. If you have a loving partner, ask him to snuggle with you. If you don't have a partner, you might find that a hot-water bottle is an acceptable substitute.

Back massage

A back rub, in which your partner squeezes the pressure away from the base of your spine *(see page 77)* may be invaluable. But don't forget the golden rule, which is to give your partner feedback, telling him what feels good and what does not.

Light touch

When a firm touch feels uncomfortable, ask your partner to try a light, fingertip touch, which might float over your skin and transform the tension into eroticism. If your discomfort is metamorphosed in this way, lovemaking and orgasm may well be therapeutic. But be aware that sometimes even a light touch can be irritating.

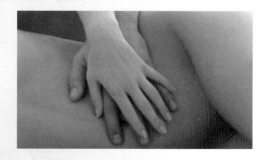

Pregnancy

Pregnancy is a time of major change for the expectant couple, above all for their relationship. As the woman grows larger, her partner sees her as a mother and this can sometimes be difficult to deal with.

Loving touch

One of the most important practical moves that a man and his partner can make at this time is literally to stay in touch. Loving touch reinforces the bonds between the partners, to their mutual benefit, but it is doubly important to the pregnant woman.

Massage during pregnancy is an excellent addition to everyday touching, cuddling, and kissing as a means of maintaining the loving bonds between a couple. Most of the strokes used in ordinary massage will also work well for pregnant women, but some of them are especially pleasing.

Back massage

By massaging her lower back, you can help to relieve the strain caused by the extra load she is carrying.

Massage strokes

The base of the spine becomes desperate for relief when it's carrying an extra load. An alternative to an ordinary back massage (*see left*) is for the woman to sit or kneel while her partner rubs her lower back gently but firmly with the palm of his hand.

A woman's legs also take the extra weight of the baby and by the end of the pregnancy they can become full of fluid. Cramping is also common, and the classic draining strokes for the legs (*see pages 101–05*) are ideal here.

The classic circling stroke (*see page 77*) can be used on all areas of the body, and fingertip strokes that brush the pregnant abdomen will stimulate the nerves on the surface of the skin and alleviate strain. When used during labor, stroking the abdomen can reduce the sensation of the contractions for some women.

After the birth

Physical and emotional problems can make this a time when it is easy for the couple to feel alienated from each other. Anything that can

---

> ## MASSAGE IN PREGNANCY
> - When massaging a pregnant woman, ask for feedback to find out which spots to focus on and which to avoid
> - Avoid putting any weight on or around the "bump"
> - The mother-to-be needs to lie down in such a way that the "bump" feels comfortable and supported
> - Ordinary back massage strokes cannot, however, be used to relieve the tension, for fear of crushing the baby.

---

build a bridge between them is therefore of great value. Touch can be such a bridge and massage a large part of the supporting structure. The touch needs to be one-way during this time—in her direction. But she can repay him later with some very special sexual treats when her desire and energy have returned.

To ease your partner's tired muscles and help her to relax, give her a soothing back massage and finish off with neck strokes, forehead circling, and a temple press (*see below*).

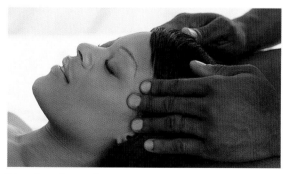

Forehead circling
Using the pads of your fingers, make tiny, circular strokes all over her forehead. Work from one side to the other and back again, varying the pressure/speed of the strokes.

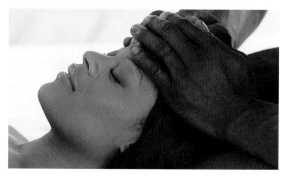

Temple press
Place your palms on each side of the forehead so that your fingers just meet. Hold your hands lightly, press gently, then hold lightly again before lifting off.

As men age

The decline in a man's sexual powers as he grows older is a rather different life change to the others in this chapter, such as menopause (*see pages 148–49*), because it is a gradual process rather than a single, identifiable event. Every man experiences it differently, but there do seem to be common denominators, both emotional and physical, that many men share.

A man of 50 will probably need twice the penile touching and rubbing to stay erect and achieve an orgasm as a man of 30. He may find that loss of hardness is a problem, as is loss of ejaculatory power and sensation. Whereas a boy of 17 will probably suffer from unwanted erections, the older man may need a lot of attention from a loving and skillful partner before he can get an erection. He may also find one orgasm a day is his limit, possibly considerably less. Sex can be compared to riding a bicycle: in good health, you can do it at any age, but you may take longer to arrive and have to pedal harder when you are older. But the journey is perhaps more pleasant if you don't rush, and the older lover can be the most satisfying.

We now know that perhaps 60 to 70 percent of impotence cases have physical causes. The majority of these are curable, so a man who becomes impotent should seek medical advice.

Hormonal changes

Although there is no hormonal menopause for men as there is for women, there is usually a gradual decline in the levels of the male sex hormone testosterone circulating in the bloodstream. Men reach their sexual peak at about the age of 18: their ability to be sexual, to feel desire, and to experience satisfactory erection and orgasm are on the decline ever after. This isn't as tough as it sounds, though, because this sexual decline is very gradual, and most middle-aged men are capable of powerful sensuality and wonderful orgasms— in the right circumstances. But most middle-aged men would probably agree that it takes longer to reach orgasm and that they need firmer direct stimulation.

Aside from declining testosterone levels, there are other aspects of aging that can affect sexual performance. Failure to achieve or maintain an erection, late-onset noninsulin-dependent diabetes, and the after-effects of prostate surgery are all instances of physical conditions that can impede the ability to have intercourse. Most men see their sexuality as an integral part of their personalities, and so they worry about such symptoms of aging.

A little help

If easy erections are vital to your confidence, the new drugs (such as Viagra, Uprima, and Cialis) work wonders.

An aging man's long-term partner may, of course, recognize that lovemaking isn't what it used to be and may encourage him to seek specialist advice. But very often, the pattern of a declining love life seems written in stone, and it takes a shift in mind-set to realize that sexual patterns can and should be altered. Be aware that you are still capable of learning new lovemaking techniques, even after 25 years of the same routine.

With a new partner, the anxious male may feel under a little pressure and consider it a burden to explain that he is not able to be as spontaneous as a young man. Most women, however, are highly tolerant of such differences and will often see new sexual needs as a challenge. If a man makes lyrical love to his partner with his hands and tongue, bringing her up to and through a series of climaxes, she isn't going to mind too much about any sex aids or special attention he subsequently needs. Instead, she is going to be more than willing to do anything she can to help his fulfillment.

Be fearless
Open your mind to making new moves to improve lovemaking.

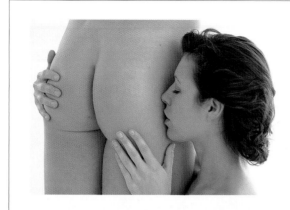

INCREASING HIS RESPONSE

• Oral sex, genital massage, and masturbation with a firm hand are good starting points. Ask him for feedback. How might you increase the feeling? Could your strokes be rougher and harder?

• What about other aspects of increasing his arousal? Would using an element of fantasy be helpful *(see pages 120–21)?*

• Anal rimming, where you run your fingertip around just inside the rim of his anus, can be extremely arousing.

"For many older couples, lovemaking can actually improve thanks to experience and wisdom."

Menopause

All women go through menopause, but although not all of them experience a midlife crisis, this can be a difficult stage in a woman's life. Just when physical changes in the body are making a woman feel older, more tired, and less attractive, not to mention anxious or depressed, children leave home and so, sometimes, do husbands.

Many women feel totally unwanted as a result of going through menopause. But on the credit side, some women feel healthier and more balanced emotionally than they have in years, and go on to tackle careers or courses of study with renewed vigor. Many couples greatly enjoy life together without the constant demands of a family, and rediscover each other as a result.

However, physical changes may make sex less satisfactory. For example, lower levels of the hormone estrogen in the menopausal woman can lead to a lessening of vaginal lubrication. She may then find intercourse uncomfortable, and also that stimulation of her genitals doesn't work as effectively as before: postmenopausal women often need longer and more careful stimulation before they can climax. Hormone replacement therapy (HRT) and lubricants and pessaries can be very effective in overcoming this.

Libido and depression

Lack of sexual desire also becomes apparent after menopause. Research shows that lovemaking often halts at around or after this time, at the instigation of the woman. One theory has it that as estrogen levels wane in the menopausal woman so, too, do levels of testosterone, the hormone that many believe is responsible for libido. Many menopausal women treated with extra testosterone report increased sexual drive, with the advantage of also experiencing increased energy and strength.

During this major life change, women need their partners to be especially understanding. A useful rule that every man should remember is this: when your partner seems abnormally volatile, ask yourself what may be going on inside her. Because the volatility may be directed toward you, it can be hard not to take it personally, but looking for other motives is always sensible.

One of the underlying characteristics of menopause can be mild depression, so mild that many women are unaware of it. But depression accentuates emotions, and acts of kindness will assume greater meaning. Giving a partner the treat of a massage, or simply arranging to do something that is for her pleasure alone, becomes a loving act of great significance.

FOR HER PLEASURE

Give her an all-over body massage, performed simply but sensitively. Ask if there are any spots of tension or pain, and try to stroke them away. Then extend the massage to her genitals, but use a vaginal lubricant (not massage oil). Use genital massage strokes *(see pages 112–13)* to build up her sexual response.

Reapply the lubricant. Let her feel bathed in it as your fingers explore first her labia and then her clitoris. Establish a rhythm, and make it clear that you are going to keep this up for a long time.

Although it may take a menopausal woman longer to climax, when she does so, it is likely to be powerful because of the extended build-up. You can also use a vibrator, but ensure that plenty of lubricant is applied.

Giving reassurance

A sense of warmth and closeness is an invaluable gift to give to a menopausal partner, and will calm and reassure her.

Sensation blockers

Both men and women are likely to experience a loss of sexual desire
and performance at some time in their lives and this can be caused
by a number of factors. While some instigators, such as depression,
are common to both sexes, others are specific to each gender.

Depression inhibits the sexual desire of males
and females. Manic depression in its manic
state often greatly exaggerates sexuality, leading
to promiscuity. Drugs and psychotherapy are
both valuable tools to overcome the condition.
The drugs used to treat schizophrenia affect
sexuality, although the condition itself does not.

Antidepressant drugs have mixed effects on
sensuality. They may bring back desire and
sensual sensation after these have been
dampened down by depression, but they also
tend to impair the mechanics of orgasm. It is
usually only by coming off antidepressants that
a person can get his or her sexual desire, arousal,
and performance fully back to normal again.

Case histories

I have come across a number of instances where
couples have had sexual problems due to one
partner experiencing either an adverse reaction
to medication they are taking or to a hormonal
imbalance. In the case of Steve, his interest in
sex with his partner, Naomi, was on the wane,
and sometimes he could not even get an
erection. When I asked him about his general
health, he said that he had been taking an ulcer-
healing preparation. I was able to reassure him
that impaired sexual function was a common
effect of the drug, and that when he had
completed the course of treatment, his libido
and potency would soon return.

In another example, Jo had a good relationship
with her boyfriend, but she was not able to
climax. Then one day, when stimulating herself
with a vibrator, she noticed that her vagina was
contracting. She was having an orgasm, but she
couldn't feel it. Jo was one of the small number
of women who have perfectly ordinary tactile
reactions to touch, but are genitally anesthetized.
We don't know why this should be, but it may
be the result of having too little free testosterone
in the bloodstream.

Providing support

If your partner is experiencing problems, let him or her know that you understand and listen sympathetically if they want to talk about it.

Female sensation blockers

Not nearly enough research has been carried out into women's sexual problems. While some are well researched, others, especially those with possible hormonal causes, need further study. But most sex researchers now agree that hormone imbalances may be a cause of sexual difficulties.

The hormone estrogen, in the right balance, is responsible for a woman's sense of well-being. It keeps the skin moist and its texture firm.

If natural estrogen dwindles, the skin becomes less elastic. Intimate touch, which formerly was pleasurable, may become irritating or even painful. The vagina is among the areas affected, and it may lose enough moisture and elasticity to make intercourse difficult without extra lubrication, and make it hard to achieve orgasm.

Testosterone, which women possess in much smaller amounts than men, provides (we think) the ability to experience sexual sensation and desire. If the level of free-ranging testosterone circulating in the blood dwindles, women lose interest in sex, may not be so eager to be touched, and find it harder to climax.

Another problem is that high levels of the hormone prolactin, which is secreted during breastfeeding, can sometimes persist after nursing has ceased. High amounts are responsible for weight

Talk it through
If a medical or emotional problem is impairing your enjoyment of sex, discuss it honestly with your partner.

gain, tiredness, and loss of interest in sex. If you experience persistent loss of sexual sensation, ask your doctor to test your hormone levels.

Illness

Most of the illnesses that affect male sexual sensation (*see pages 154–55*) will also affect women, but there are some that women are more prone to. Older women who have not been on hormone replacement therapy (HRT) may find that their joints ache and, later, that they suffer from osteoporosis, or "brittle bones." "Dowager's hump," the stoop caused by the crumbling of the top of the spine, is one result of this condition.

Pain in arthritic hips is much more common in women with osteoporosis, and pain in the joints makes lovemaking difficult. If a woman begins HRT in her mid to late 40s, it will act as a preventative to osteoporosis. Older women benefit from starting HRT because it can restore bone density to some extent. It also gives some protection against heart attack.

Just as male sexual activity is made possible by a healthy blood supply to the penis, female sexual activity is similarly facilitated. Although research is limited, it's reasonable to assume that just as obstructions to the blood supply in this area affect male erection, they are equally likely to impair female sexual response. Arterial disease might be responsible, and so might scar tissue.

Studies of diabetic women have shown them to be free of sexual problems, provided that their diabetes is well controlled. They are, however, more prone to vaginal infections such as yeast infections. And, of course, sexual infections of any sort disrupt a good sexual experience and always require prompt medical treatment.

THE EFFECTS OF SURGERY

Anesthesia and the shock of surgery may cause depression, which in turn lowers desire for sex. Talking feelings through can help, but in most cases the depression lifts spontaneously anyway. Some radical surgery such as a mastectomy or stoma surgery may prove extremely depressing, but loving touch can restore good spirits and good sensation.

Ovariohysterectomy (removal of the uterus, fallopian tubes, and ovaries) has a more extreme effect. Regardless of age, women experience its after-effects as menopause, and this may be accompanied by the classic signs, including vaginal dryness. Hormone replacement therapy (HRT) and estrogen cream for the vagina can be a great help.

Vaginal surgery, tears during childbirth and their subsequent repair, and surgery affecting the rectum may all inhibit perineal blood supply, with the effect of reducing sexual response. Poor stitching after childbirth can make intercourse painful, but can be remedied by surgery to cut out the scar tissue.

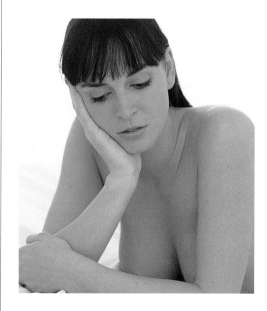

Male sensation blockers

I remember feeling puzzled, early in my massage studies, by occasionally coming across men who seemed to get little real enjoyment out of my tactile attentions. Yes, the sensation was pleasant, they'd concede, but it wasn't anything particularly special. The men who said this were invariably the possessors of what felt like very solid flesh. Whenever I gave such a man a massage, I couldn't move his skin in ripples because it seemed to be fastened to one place. It felt to me as though powerful muscles were quite literally blocking the action of my hands, and also blocking any sensation for him. It wasn't until I read about Wilhelm Reich's concept of "body armor" that I gained some insight into this problem. Reich's theory is that some people are permanently tense, and that this tension is expressed by unconsciously holding the muscles taut. The overall effect is that the tense person is wearing a layer of muscular armor to protect himself from the intrusions of the outside world.

What were the repercussions of this for making love, I wondered? Common sense told me that such a man would probably get little out of overall body contact and would instead be likely to focus all his sensuality on his penis, the one organ allowed to be "vulnerable." I checked this out by asking these men, and they agreed.

The answer offered by many professional masseurs is "rolfing." This is a form of very deep massage, invented by Dr. Ida Rolf of Colorado. It is painful to receive, and when offered is usually combined with talking therapy: as the tension decreases, the person being massaged talks about what may have contributed to building up such barriers. Rolfing isn't a

PHYSICAL SENSATION BLOCKERS

Diseases that affect the nerves, such as multiple sclerosis, can reduce tactile sensation. Some localized conditions also affect sexual response; nerve damage after prostate operations may cause inability to achieve erections. Other causes of dysfunction are pain from arthritis and anxiety as a result of asthma, which can result in the unconscious blocking of sexual signals from the brain to the genitals.

Surgery can create mild depression, which may in turn result in lessened sexual desire for a while. For some men even the suggestion that surgery can impair their sexual feeling may cause a loss of feeling. A positive attitude often reduces the risk of this happening. Finally, diabetes affects erection but not desire; here, injection therapy can provide artificial erections.

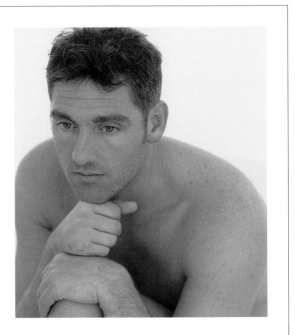

technique that can be done by amateur masseurs and it is best left to the professionals.

Drugs

Other causes of male sensation blockers might be adverse reactions to certain drugs. Many of the drugs commonly used in the prevention and cure of illness can impair sexual performance, as can alcohol and illicit "recreational" drugs such as cocaine (*see pages 156–57*). Alcohol is a brain depressant. In small amounts, it reduces anxiety and inhibition, and this may allow sexy feelings to emerge that otherwise would not be given

the chance. In larger doses, however, alcohol rapidly impairs physical and mental functions, including sexual response, in both men and women. It reduces testosterone levels, and many men find it difficult to get an erection when they are drunk. Barbiturates and other hypnotic drugs have a similar action.

Reassuring touch

Use warmth moves, such as stroking and squeezing, to reassure your partner.

Sexual effects of drugs

A great many of the medicines prescribed for common medical problems can have unwanted sexual side-effects. In addition, while some medicines may not possess any unpleasant side-effects when taken on their own, side-effects may appear if the drugs are combined with alcohol or with other medicines. It is vital, therefore, that you check all drug usage beforehand with your doctor or pharmacist.

ALCOHOL

Small amounts may increase sexual desire by reducing anxiety and loosening inhibitions. Moderate amounts can impair a man's ability to achieve or sustain an erection and may prevent him from ejaculating; chronic alcohol abuse can make a man impotent.

ANABOLIC STEROIDS

Such as nandrolone. Misuse of these drugs can cause a number of sexual problems, some of which are serious. In men, these include a drop in the amount of the sex hormone testosterone circulating in the blood, leading to decreased sexual desire; shrinkage of the testicles; impaired sperm production; and growth of the breasts. Women may grow facial and body hair and develop male-pattern baldness, and experience menstrual and ovulation problems and enlargement of the clitoris. Steroid misuse can also trigger rapid mood swings, increased aggressiveness, paranoia, and psychosis.

ANTIDEPRESSANTS

Tricyclics, such as amitriptyline; **selective serotonin reuptake inhibitors (SSRIs)**, such as fluoxetine; **monoamine-oxidase inhibitors (MAOIs)**, such as phenelzine.
Antidepressants may cause a loss of libido, an inability to achieve orgasm in both men and women, and failure in men to achieve an erection.

BLOOD-PRESSURE CONTROL DRUGS (ANTIHYPERTENSIVES)

Beta-blockers, such as propranolol; **alpha-blockers**, such as doxazosin.
Some antihypertensives can cause erection problems in men.

CANNABIS

Reports of the sexual effects of small amounts are very subjective and difficult to quantify, but one of the main effects of the drug appears to be an enhancement of the user's state of mind. For example, if you are feeling tired, it will send you to sleep; if you are feeling sexy, it can make you feel more so. The effects of heavy long-term use are more serious but usually disappear quickly when consumption ceases. Effects include a drop in the amount of the sex hormone testosterone circulating in the blood, leading to decreased sexual desire; impotence and impaired sperm production (men); and impaired ovarian function (women).

COCAINE

Small amounts may increase sexual desire and enable men to delay orgasm, but prolonged heavy use can lead to sexual dysfunction in both men (impotence) and women (orgasmic failure).

DIURETICS

Thiazides, such as bendrofluazide.
Sexual problems may affect a small percentage of people taking these drugs: desire may be reduced, and some men develop erection problems.
Potassium-sparing diuretics, such as spironolactone.
These drugs can cause a decrease in sexual desire and erection problems for men.

H2-RECEPTOR ANTAGONISTS (IN ULCER-HEALING PREPARATIONS)

Such as cimetidine and ranitidine.
These drugs can, on rare occasions, cause erection problems in men.

HORMONAL PREPARATIONS

Androgens, such as testosterone preparations. These drugs may help to restore sex drive and orgasmic ability in both men and women.
Antiandrogens, such as cyproterone acetate. Reduced sexual desire may occur in both men and women; men may also experience erection problems.
Estrogens These hormones may improve vaginal lubrication in postmenopausal women, but in men they can cause loss of sexual desire and erection problems.
Oral contraceptives The effects appear very variable: some women find that sexual desire decreases, others that it increases (perhaps because these drugs ensure that intercourse does not lead to pregnancy).

NARCOTICS

Diamorphine hydrochloride (*heroin*), **methadone hydrochloride** (*methadone, Physeptone*)
Short-term use can lead to decreased sexual desire, and addiction in men often leads to impotence, ejaculation problems, and sterility. Female addicts may lose the ability to orgasm.

SLEEPING PREPARATIONS

Such as nitrazepam. Some sleeping drugs are associated with changes in libido.

TRANQUILLIZERS

Benzodiazepines, including lorazepam, chlordiazepoxide, diazepam, clorazepate, dipotassium. Use can lead to loss of libido.
Phenothiazines, such as chlorpromazine hydrochloride; **butyrophenones**, such as benperidol.
May cause erection problems in men.

Index

A

abuse, history of 14–15
aging
  male 144–47
  and menopause 148–49,
   153
  sex and 109, 118, 138–39
alcohol 155–56
anabolic steroids 156
antidepressants 150, 156

B

Barbach, Lonnie 125
bathing and showering 38,
  41, 126, 131
blood-pressure control drugs
  156

C

cannabis 156
climax see orgasm
clitoris 61, 63–65, 135, 149
  clitoral maneuvers 110,
   113
clothing, choice of 21, 23
cocaine 155–56

D

depression 18, 148, 150, 153
diabetes 144, 153
Dodson, Betty 125
drainage see massage,
  lymphatic
drugs 155–57
  see also medical conditions

E

erogenous zones 44–53,
  60–63, 77, 129
  see also female; intimate
  massage; male;
  questionnaire, Sexual body

eroticism 108–09, 141
exercises
  arm 31
  dressmaker's dummy 30–33
  head tilting 30–31
  leg 32
  magic mirror 39
  massage, before 24–25
  myotonic 59
  relaxation 22, 25, 141
  self-help 39
  "third eye" 27
  waist lifts 32–33
  see also massage; touch

F

fantasy and sex 68–69,
  118–21, 147
female
  clitoris see clitoris
  desire, loss of 150–53
  erogenous zones see
   erogenous zones
  G-spot 135
  genital stimulation 61–63
  hormone levels 69, 140,
   148, 150–53
  intimate massage see
   intimate massage
  lesbians 60–61, 63
  libido 119, 139, 148
  masturbation 69, 109, 119,
   135
  menopause 148–49
  menstruation 140–41
  nipples see nipples
  orgasm 57, 61, 64–67, 121,
   125, 150, 152
  orgasm, multiple 67–69
  pregnancy 142–43,
   153
  resolution phase 67

self-touch massage 124–25,
  130–35, 150
sensuality 60–63
sex flush 64–66
sexual response 64–67
  vagina 57, 61, 64–65,
   148–49
  vaginal secretions 61, 64
  vibrators 135, 148, 150
Fithian, Marilyn 46, 58

G

games
  dressmaker's dummy 30–33
  hair sweep 38–39
  massage 26–29, 38–41
  shampooing 26–29
  touch 16–19
  see also massage; touch
genitals see intimate massage

H

Hartman, William 46, 58
hormone levels
  female 69, 140, 148, 150–53
  male 144, 155
hormone preparations 157

I

impotence 144–47
incense 75
Institute for the Advanced
  Study of Human Sexuality
  6–7, 110
intimate massage
  clitoral maneuvers 110, 113
  corkscrew 117
  countdown 115
  duck's bill 110, 113
  and eroticism 108–09, 121,
   141
  female 48, 110–13, 135

G-spot 135
gentle hair torture 110, 112
hand over hand 117
lemon squeezer 117
male 114–17, 129
squeeze technique 117
wibbling 110, 113
see also erogenous zones;
  sex

K

Kaplan, Dr. Helen Singer 67
Kinsey, Alfred 54–57
Konnoff, Nick 59

M

male
  aging 144–47
  and desire, loss of 150–55
  ejaculation 52, 56–59, 69,
   117
  erection 54, 59, 119,
   144–47
  homosexuality 52–55
  hormone levels 144, 155
  impotence 144–47
  intimate massage see
   intimate massage
  masturbation 109, 119, 147
  myotonic exercise 59
  nipples see nipples
  orgasm 54–56, 144
  orgasm, multiple 58–59
  penile stimulation 51, 115,
   129
  refractory phase 54, 56
  self-touch massage 124–29
  sensuality 50–53
  sex flush 54, 56
  sexual response 54–57, 147
  testicles 52, 54, 59, 115,
   129

massage
  abdominal 88, 127
  arm 31, 92–95, 128, 133
  back 76–83, 141–43
  belly 87–88
  breast 47, 60–61, 64, 87,
    90–91, 133
  buttocks 49, 128, 133
  chest 46, 127
  clothing, choice of 21, 23
  for drainage *see* massage,
    lymphatic
  emotional benefits of
    17–19, 93
  exercises *see* exercises
  feedback, giving 20–21, 48,
    51, 73–75, 77, 141, 147
  foot 34–37, 75, 105, 132
  front 84–89
  games *see* games
  ground rules, establishing
    20–21
  guidelines, basic 21
  hand 41, 75, 93, 96–99, 128
  head 26–29, 44, 84–85, 143
  intimate *see* intimate
    massage
  joy of 72–75
  leg 46, 49, 100–05, 129,
    134, 143
  lymphatic 93, 95, 101, 105,
    143
  and medical conditions 21
  nipple *see* nipples
  oil 23, 39, 75, 78, 84, 110,
    113
  and pregnancy 142–43
  preparation for 22–25,
    73–75, 77
  rolfing 155–56
  rules, ten golden 73
  self-touch 124–35
  shoulder 75, 83, 84
  and stress relief 19
  strokes *see* strokes, massage
  and surroundings, sensual
    23, 75, 132
  thigh 46, 128, 134
  toe 37, 129, 132
  whole-body 73, 149
  see also touch
Masters and Johnson 51–52,
  60–61, 63, 66, 67
masturbation 69, 109, 119,
  135, 147
medical conditions
  and massage 21
  and sexual desire 144,
    150–53
  see also drugs
music 75

N

narcotics 157
neck and shoulders 63,
  133
nipples
  and female sensuality
    64–66, 133
  and male sensuality 52, 56,
    127
  see also massage, breast

O

orgasm
  female 57, 61, 64–67, 121,
    125, 150, 152
  female, multiple 67–69
  male 54–56, 144
  male, multiple 58–59

Q

questionnaire
  Touch 13
  Touch intensity 49–51
  Sexual body 46–47, 50

R

reflexology 35
Reich, Wilhelm 154
relationship problems 11
  see also aging
relaxation 22, 25, 141
Rolf, Dr. Ida 154–55

S

sex
  and abuse 14–15
  and aging 138–39
  and desire, loss of 150–53
  and drugs 155–57
  education 45
  and fantasy 68–69,
    118–21, 147
  intercourse 20, 49
  oral 147
  see also intimate massage
showering and bathing 38,
  41, 126, 131
skin
  sensitivity 11, 47
  as sex organ 10–13
  see also erogenous zones;
    touch
sleeping preparations 157
strokes, massage
  abdominal twist 88
  anal rimming 147
  armpit stretch 95
  breast cupping 84, 87
  caterpillar 80
  circling 37, 77, 79, 87–88,
    98, 101, 143
  clawing 80
  cross-currents 79
  fairy rings 84–85
  finger lacing 97
  glide 77
  hand over hand 102, 105,
    117
  head lift 84–85
  hip lift 82
  kneading 79, 87, 92, 96,
    101, 104
  kneecapping 103–04
  knuckling 36, 97, 132
  oiling and spoiling 93, 100,
    103
  patterns of 73–75, 93, 141
  pulling 31, 94
  shoulder blade, raised
    83–85
  single hand 82
  slide 84–86, 88, 91
  spinal taps 82, 89
  temple press 27, 143
  thumbing 36, 79, 82, 83,
    98, 132
  twisting 94
  see also intimate massage
Stubbs, Ray 6–7, 110

T

ticklishness 34–35, 88, 127
touch
  and abuse, history of
14–15
  body exploration and
    44–49
  connecting through 11–12
  cultural differences 12
  emotional benefits of
    17–19
  erogenous zones *see*
    erogenous zones
  first experiences of 11–17,
    18
  games *see* games
  hair and scalp 26–29, 44
  and menstruation 140–41
  and moods, tuning into 17
  patterns 139
  questionnaires 13, 49–51,
    60
  socializing through 17
  see also massage; skin;
    strokes, massage
tranquillizers 157

U

ulcer-healing medication 157

V

vibrators 135, 148, 150

Acknowledgments

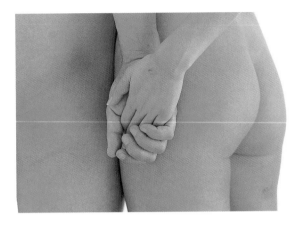

The author would like to thank:
Kenneth Ray Stubbs and the Rev. Ted McIlvenna.

Dorling Kindersley would like to thank:
Photographer: Ruth Jenkinson
Photographer's assistant: Sam White
Art director and stylist on photoshoots: Ruth Hope
For additional styling: Kerry Hope
Makeup artist: Susie Kennett
Jacket designer: Chloe Alexander
Indexer: Margaret McCormack